Small-Bowel Obstruction

Roberto Di Mizio • Mariano Scaglione

Small-Bowel Obstruction

CT Features with Plain Film and US Correlations

Springer

Editors

Roberto Di Mizio
Chief, Radiology Department
"San Massimo" Hospital
Penne (PE)
Italy

Mariano Scaglione
Chief, Emergency and Trauma CT Section
Department of Diagnostic Imaging
"A. Cardarelli" Hospital
Naples
Italy

Originally published as:
Ileo meccanico dell'intestino tenue
Aspetti TC e correlazioni eco-radiografiche
a cura di Roberto Di Mizio e Mariano Scaglione

Translated by the Editors with friendly collaboration of Otto Chan, M.D., Consultant Radiologist, London Independent Hospital, UK
Drawings by: Veronica Di Mizio, Chieti

ISBN 978-88-470-5622-0 Springer Milan Berlin Heidelberg New York
ISBN 978-88-470-0667-6 (eBook)
Springer is part of Springer Science+Business Media
springer.com

Softcover re-print of the Hardcover 1st edition 2007

Cover layout: Simona Colombo, Milan, Italy
Typesetting: Compostudio, Cernusco s/N (Milan), Italy
Printing: Arti Grafiche Nidasio, Assago (Milan), Italy

Springer-Verlag Italia S.r.l., Via Decembrio 28, I-20137 Milan, Italy

Foreword to the English Edition

Intestinal obstruction is often a daunting topic for both radiologists and surgeons. The varying manifestations of luminal blockage of the large and small bowel at initial presentation and upon recurrence, the range of clinical signs and symptoms, and the limited helpful laboratory data sometimes make diagnosis difficult, even when the occlusion is uncomplicated. The issue becomes even more complex when complications such as strangulation and infarction ensue. The proliferation of imaging studies in the last two decades has enhanced our capability to diagnose bowel obstruction in all its manifestations. Yet at the same time, it has engendered confusion when trying to determine the most appropriate protocol in various circumstances. Its advocates often trumpet the virtues of each test. However, the proper sequencing of tests, beyond the plain film, has received less consideration and little consensus from experts in the field.

This monograph presents exquisite depictions of the various manifestations of intestinal obstruction as demonstrated by radiography, ultrasonography and computed tomography. The images are crisp, clear and pertinent. Only the most up-to-date equipment is used to produce revealing images, all of which are supplemented by apt legends. The discussions are concise and illuminating. This monograph will be a valuable addition to the referential armamentarium that is essential for any radiologist dealing with emergency and other acute conditions.

Practice patterns in various English-speaking countries vary greatly in the assessment of intestinal obstruction. From reading of many publications on the topic, I can say there is no one correct way to evaluate these conditions. The availability of imaging studies and historical information, pertinent laboratory data, biases of individual interpreters and skill or lack of available ultrasonographers allows for a range of diagnostic protocols to be employed for rapid determination of intestinal obstruction and its ancillary manifestations. Therefore, this book will best be used as a guide, not as a bible. Regardless of how individual radiologists and surgeons use this book, it will be most helpful in illustrating and describing the various manifestations of this frequently challenging diagnosis.

Newark, July 2007

Stephen R. Baker, MD
Professor and Chairman
Department of Radiology
University of Medicine and Dentistry of New Jersey
New Jersey Medical School
Newark, NJ, USA

Foreword to the Italian Edition

This book comes from a great distance... from the deep knowledge and extensive experience acquired on a daily basis by a group of radiologists highly attentive to the pathophysiology and morphodynamic aspects of the small bowel and acute abdomen. Through correct interpretation of imaging findings of small-bowel obstruction, the radiologist affords the physician the possibility of reaching not only the correct diagnosis but also of defining the exact chronology of this event, thus quickly addressing the most appropriate management for the case.

The decision to illustrate small-bowel obstruction in the form of an atlas textbook comes from the itinerant courses of the Section of Emergency Radiology of the Società Italiana di Radiologia Medica (Italian Society of Radiology). This topic has always stimulated the attention of attendees, who have often requested a simple, understandable and straightforward text that would serve as a readily available reference.

This book presents itself particularly well to this purpose, illustrating the entire spectrum of findings that every radiologist should know. Its extensive images explain the integration of plain film and sonography; nevertheless, most of the book is dedicated to the imaging of computed tomography, which is the superior imaging technique in understanding the loop-mesentery complex.

With this book, the authors fill a gap in the scientific literature on a difficult topic, which requires an in-depth knowledge of its pathophysiology in order to accurately interpret the imaging of small-bowel obstruction. I hope further, similar editorial initiatives will follow shortly.

Naples, February 2007

Prof. Roberto Grassi
President
Section of Emergency Radiology
Italian Society of Radiology

Table of Contents

List of Contributors

Simone Altobelli
Division of General Surgery
"San Massimo" Hospital
Penne (PE)
Italy

Giuseppina Annunziata
Institute of Radiology
Second University of Naples
Naples
Italy

Roberta Cianci
Department of Clinical Sciences and Bioimages
Section of Radiology
"G. D'Annunzio" University
Chieti
Italy

Maria Antonietta Colasante
Health District
ASL Pescara
Penne (PE)
Italy

Fenesia D'Amario
Radiology Service
"San Massimo" Hospital
Penne (PE)
Italy

Giampiero D'Amico
Division of General Surgery
"San Massimo" Hospital
Penne (PE)
Italy

Remo Della Marra
Radiology Department
"San Massimo" Hospital
Penne (PE)
Italy

Roberto Di Mizio
Radiology Department
"San Massimo" Hospital
Penne (PE)
Italy

Veronica Di Mizio
Department of Clinical Sciences and Bioimages
Section of Radiology
"G. D'Annunzio" University
Chieti
Italy

Dario Di Rocco
Radiology Department
"San Massimo" Hospital
Penne (PE)
Italy

Antonella Filippone
Department of Clinical Sciences and Bioimages
Section of Radiology
"G. D'Annunzio" University
Chieti
Italy

Roberto Grassi
Institute of Radiology
Second University of Naples
Naples
Italy

Paolo Innocenti
Department of Surgical Sciences
General and Laparoscopic Surgery
"G. D'Annunzio" University
Chieti
Italy

Gustavo Maggi
Division of General Surgery
"San Massimo" Hospital
Penne (PE)
Italy

Luigia Romano
Department of Diagnostic Imaging
"A. Cardarelli" Hospital
Naples
Italy

Mariano Scaglione
Emergency and Trauma CT Section
Department of Diagnostic Imaging
"A. Cardarelli" Hospital
Naples
Italy

Roberto Sciarra
Radiology Department
"San Massimo" Hospital
Penne (PE)
Italy

Introduction

Small-bowel obstruction (SBO) is responsible for about 15% of surgical operations for an acute abdomen. In Italy, the most frequent causes of SBO are adhesions (about 60%), hernias (about 20%) and neoplasms (about 15%). Comparison with other countries is interesting. In the USA, the most frequent cause of SBO is adhesional syndrome (50–75%), followed by stenosing Crohn's enteritis and neoplasms; it is interesting to note that hernias are not present due to extensive preventive measures for external hernias. On the contrary, in developing countries, hernias still account for about 78% of SBO as a consequence of the lack of preventive measures. Furthermore, due to the limited number of performed abdominal surgeries, adhesional syndrome is only responsible for 10% of the cases.

SBO is characterised by interruption of lumen continuity, with acute intestinal changes in canalisation. The obstructive site causes dilatation of intestinal loops proximal and progressive collapse of the loops distal. Intestinal stasis is always mixed: gaseous and liquid. SBO has an intrinsic dynamism: in other words, it is capable of evolutionary development.

New imaging methods have basically revolutionised the role of conventional radiology in the evaluation of the acute abdomen. Nevertheless, abdominal plain film still a role in the study of acute intestinal behaviours.

In suspected SBO, we always perform ultrasonography (US) as an integrative modality to abdominal plain film. US confirms and supports the diagnosis, offers additional, important findings and enhances overall diagnostic confidence. To date, contrast-enhanced multidetector computed tomography (MDCT) is the gold standard in the study of SBO. In the diagnostic work-up of SBO, MDCT can be performed both as the first imaging modality and as an integrative modality to US–plain film study.

Objectives of the present work are the following:

- to illustrate the mechanism of SBO;
- to connect the pathophysiology of SBO to MDCT imaging;
- to describe contrast-enhanced CT findings of SBO;
- to show the corresponding US–plain film correlations.

This work examines the issues of acute SBO in adult.

1 Formation Mechanisms

R. Di Mizio, F. D'Amario, V. Di Mizio, M.A. Colasante, G. D'Amico, G. Maggi, P. Innocenti, M. Scaglione

Various mechanisms of formation of acute small-bowel obstruction (SBO) allow the following subdivisions:

- obturation;
- narrowing;
- compression;
- blockage;
- intussusception;
- large-bowel obstruction;
- intestinal strangling and strangulation;
- complex mechanisms.

SBO by Obturation

This is caused by intestinal lumen occupation due to the obturation mechanism, which involves the lumen exclusively. The term obturation adequately emphasises the first and unique mechanism of formation of this kind of obstruction, which is due to simple occupation of the intestinal lumen. Obturation is caused by the presence of extraneous material in the gut lumen exclusively. This material may be:

- alimentary bolus (Fig. 1.1);
- gallstone migration into the intestine;
- polypoid mass originating from the stomach, duodenum and small bowel;
- foreign body.

Obstruction by obturation must be considered the prototype of simple acute obstruction, because it is caused exclusively by a blocked lumen. In this way, the mechanical effect determines alterations of the lumen and bowel wall only, without complex consequences on the loop and its mesentery and on the vascular supply.

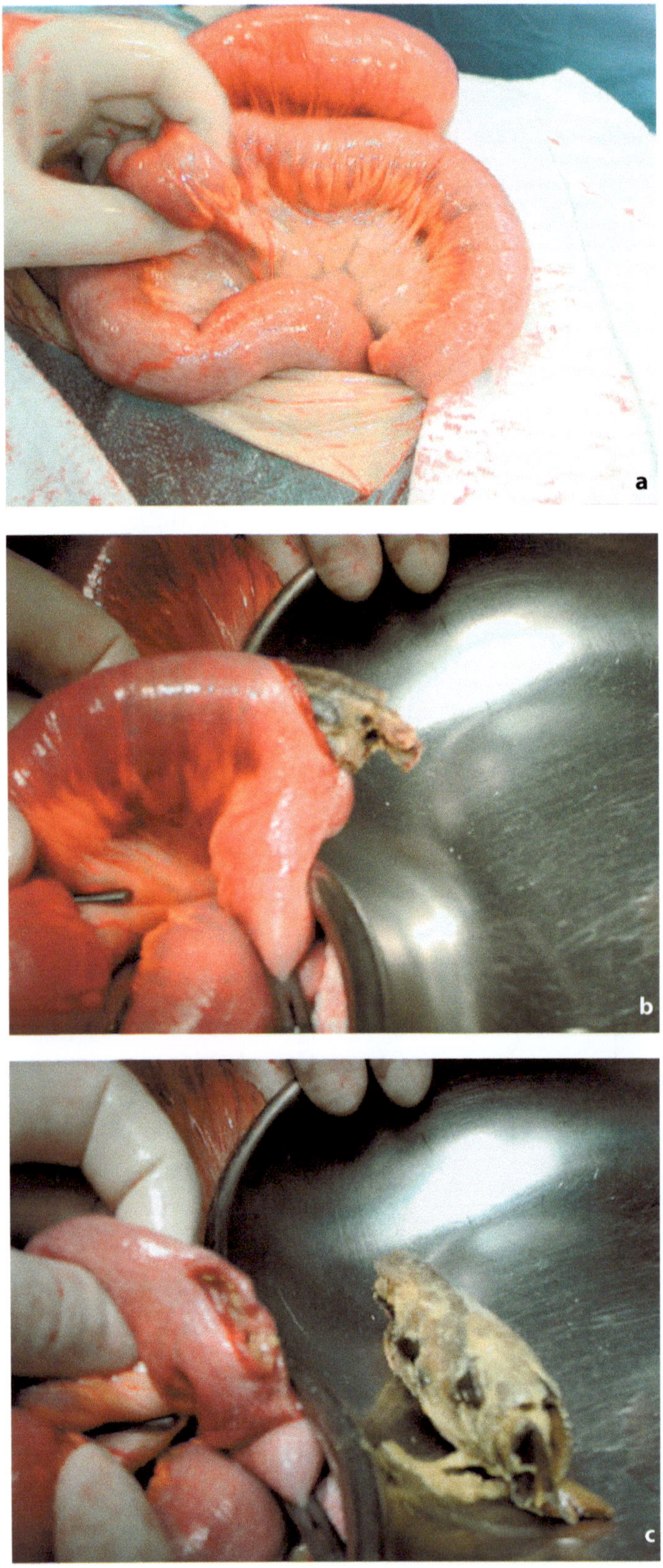

Fig. 1.1 a-c. Small-bowel obstruction by obturation. **a** The surgeon identifies obstructive bolus. Moderately dilated loops. Normal mesentery. **b**, **c** Enterotomy and phytobezoar removal

SBO by Narrowing

This type of obstruction is caused by lumen narrowing and is almost always accompanied by pathological thickening of the bowel wall. Increase in wall thickness occurs at the cost of lumen diameter, which is reduced more or less significantly.

Lumen narrowing can be caused by:

- Intramural pathological processes (inflammatory – for instance, Crohn's disease (Fig. 1.2), neoplastic or vascular diseases.
- Mesenteric retraction, which causes wall deformity and rigidity with consequent lumen narrowing. In particular, mesenteritis in Crohn's disease, post-actinic mesenteritis and retractile mesenteritis must be considered. Pathological wall thickening may not be present.
- Infiltrating and expanding processes of the abdominal cavity. These processes first compress and then infiltrate the intestinal wall, causing lumen reduction due to the mechanisms of compression and narrowing.

SBO in never serrated and persistent. Abrupt onset of intestinal obstruction is usually due to a mechanism of obturation caused by an alimentary bolus, which causes a chronic subocclusive condition. Sometimes, topographical variations in loop site and location are present.

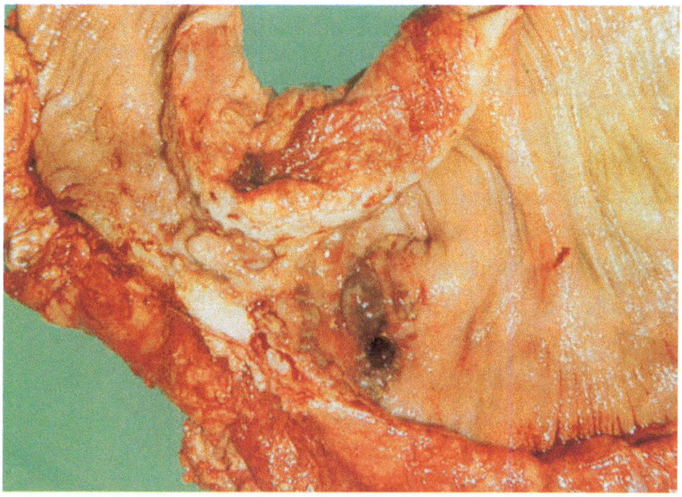

Fig. 1.2. Small-bowel obstruction by lumen narrowing. Crohn's enteritis causes marked wall thickening. Short and tight lumen stenosis with proximal dilatation. Evidence of pseudopolyps and mucosal atrophy

SBO by Compression

Lumen reduction is due to bowel-wall indentation, resulting from adjacent abdominal masses causing extrinsic compression upon the outer border of the loop. This mechanical effect may be caused, for example, by an intestinal loop trapped inside a hernia, when the hernia neck causes only bowel-wall compression without strangling.

SBO of this type is seldom serious. Topographical variations in loop site and location may occur.

SBO by Blockage

The mechanism of this type of SBO is supported by extrinsic pathological entities, such as adhesional bands, adhesions and perivisceritis, which subtend the loop surface, causing compression and collapse (Figs. 1.3 and 1.4). In geometry, the term subtend defines the rectilinear segment, called the cord, which joins the end points of an arch. In this particular type of SBO, the arch corresponds to the loop and the cord to the adhesional band. A high-grade obstruction is often caused by the coexistence of angulation or loop torsion. If the mechanism of blockage acts significantly at two points of the arch created by the bowel loop, the result is a closed-loop obstruction.

Approximately 90% of patients who have undergone abdominal surgery present with abdominal adhesions following laparotomy. In most cases, adhesional bands are not responsible for bowel obstruction. Causes of mechanical blockage in SBO are adhesions following abdominal surgery (80%), congenital or inflammatory bands (10%) and idiopathic bands (10%).

Blockage by Adhesional Band

An adhesional band causes a serrated fulcrum point: complete lumen blockage causes sudden and rapid distension of bowel loops. Topographic location of the small bowel generally respects the natural arrangement of small-bowel loops along the mesenteric root. Prompt surgical evaluation is indicated in this type of obstruction.

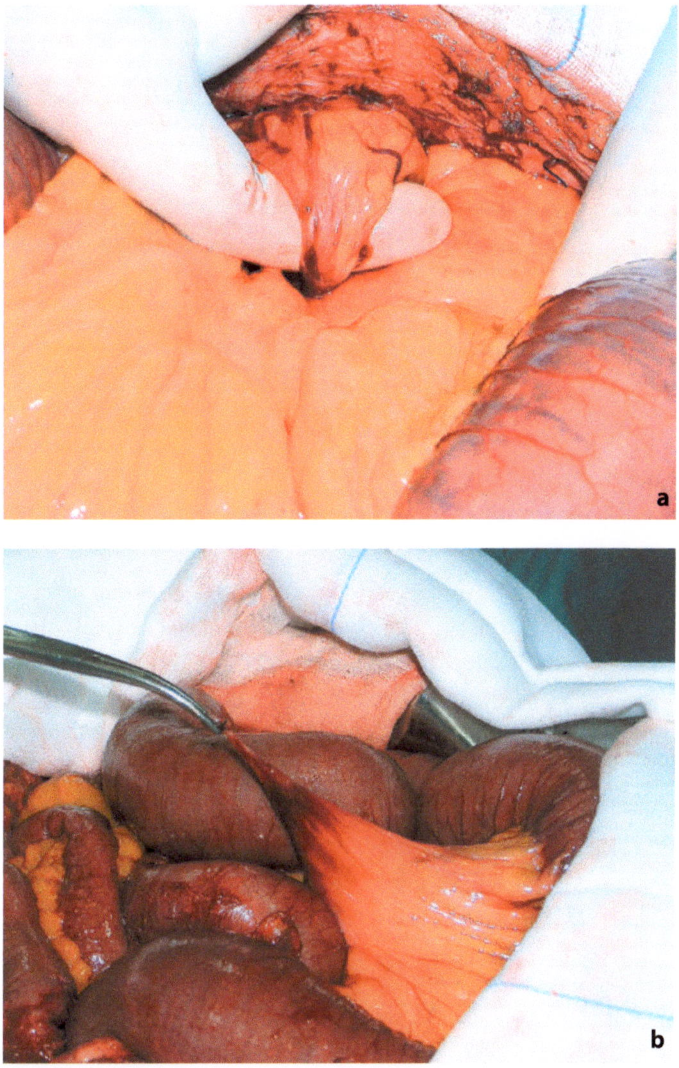

Fig. 1.3 a, b. Small-bowel obstruction by blockage. Wide adhesional band of the mesentery is surgically isolated (**a**) and resected (**b**). Proximal loops to the obstructive band are dilated. Distal loops are collapsed. Normal mesentery

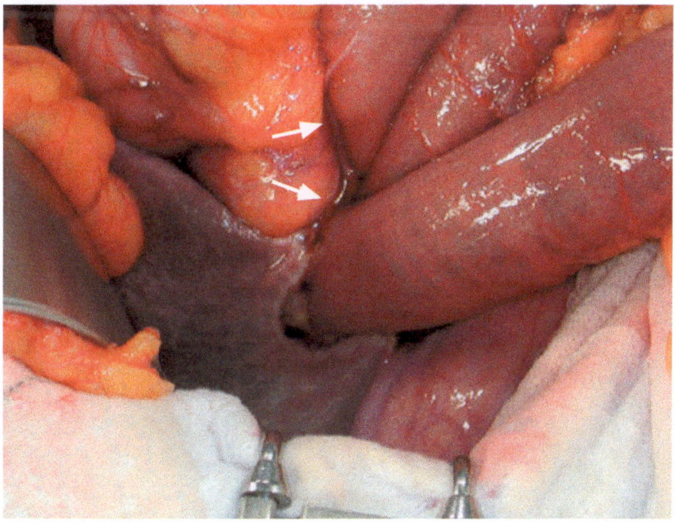

Fig. 1.4. Small-bowel obstruction by blockage. At the level of the inferior margin of the liver, a thin band (*arrows*) subtends the loop surface, causing compression and collapse. Proximal dilated loops

Blockage by Tenting Adhesions

Tenting adhesion obstruction generally has a gradual evolution. Acute obstruction is very often due to fixation and angulation of bowel loops, causing asymmetric and partial luminal reduction. Alimentary bolus impaction causes progression to complete luminal obstruction.

This may be complicated by tenting adhesions formed between two or more adjacent small-bowel loops or fixation of loops to the anterior abdominal wall and/or other abdominal organs. Neoperitoneal cavities, defining situations such as that of internal hernia, may be formed. This explains frequent changes of topographic arrangement and location of the small bowel. Fibrin deposition can mimic adhesive causes (Fig. 1.5).

Blockage by Extensive Adhesions

SBO caused by extensive adhesions occurs as an acute consequence of chronic perivisceral processes. Multiple adhesions aggregate loops and frequently anchor to the mesentery. These conditions tend to form complex images; they produce chronic subocclusive images leading to recurrent and swinging episodes.

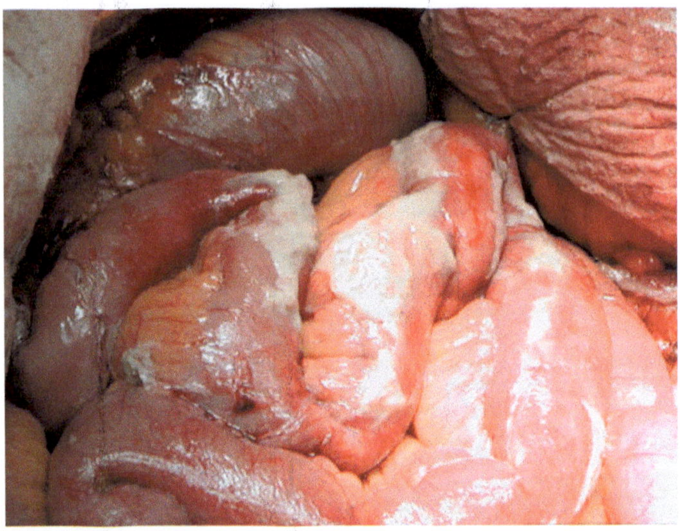

Fig. 1.5. Small-bowel obstruction by fibrin. Considerable amount of fibrin mimics adhesional phenomena with multiple loop angulations. There is intestinal distension and absence of peritoneal fluid

SBO by Intussusception

Intussusception is a situation in which part of the intestine (intussusceptum) has prolapsed into an adjacent tract of intestine (intussuscipiens), causing lumen obstruction. It is an unusual cause of small-bowel obturation. Intussusception corresponds to telescopic herniating involvement of one portion of the intestine into an adjacent one, like one part of a telescope sliding into itself. In other words, it consists of intestinal hernia into the intestine (Fig. 1.6).

In adult, a definite cause is identifiable in about 92% of cases, and is idiopathic in 8%. Typically, intussusception is due to polypoid lesions; it may be also occur as a complication of celiac disease or by an invaginated Meckel's diverticulum. In adult, intussusception must be considered as a complication of neoplastic diseases.

On the basis of consequences on canalisation, three different types of intussusception are identifiable.

Cold Intussusception

This indicates an asymptomatic clinical picture, without abdominal pain and obstructive symptoms. This presentation, although infrequent, is little known but not uncommon; intussusception is often enteroenteric and requires careful diagnostic evaluation.

Incomplete and Reversible Hot Intussusception

This is intussusception with a mild degree of obstruction without vascular changes. The invaginating tract may resolve spontaneously, although this condition is likely to be recurrent. This type of invagination causes recurrent and transient episodes of intestinal obstruction.

Complete and Irreversible Hot Intussusception

This kind of intussusception implies simultaneous involvement of a bowel segment and its vascular supply. It is a particular type of strangling hernia prolapsed into the intestine. It forms a stable obstruction with progressive vascular insufficiency. This type of complicated invagination may have dramatic clinical implications and evolution, as it involves neurovascular components of the bowel–mesentery system and visceral serosa.

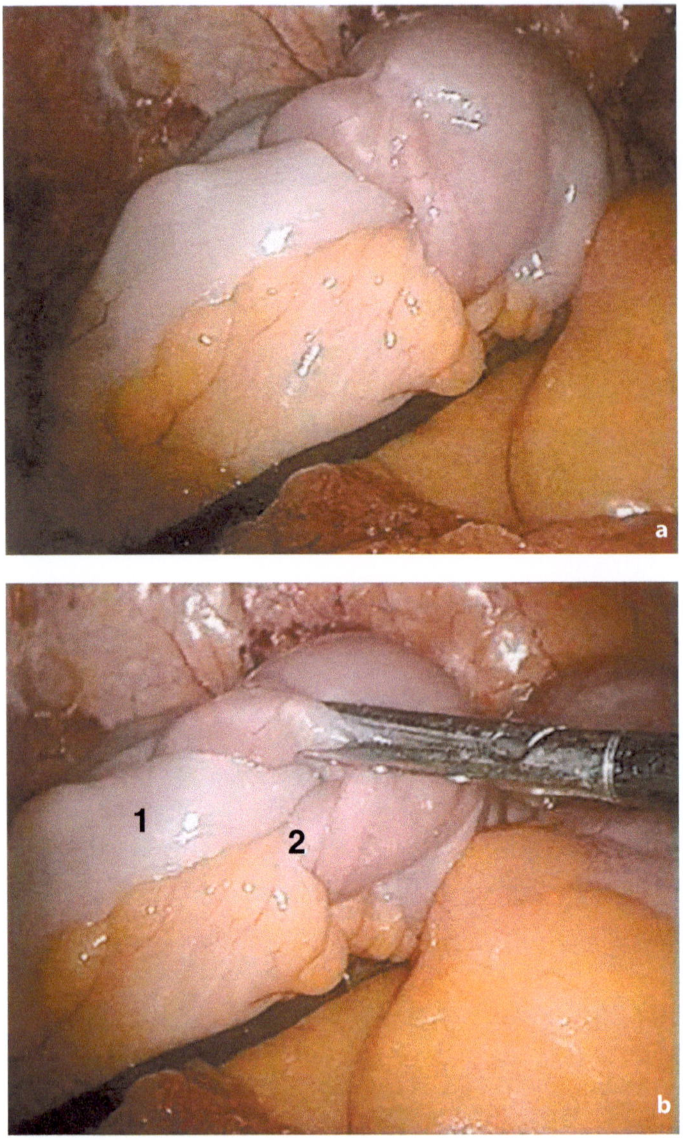

Fig. 1.6 a-d. Enteroenteric intussusception. Videolaparoscopic operation. **a** An intestinal tract is invaginated into an adjacent distal loop carrying its mesentery. The intestinal wall and mesentery appear normal. There is absence of dilatation of invaginated loop (cold intussusception). **b** The surgeon raises the invaginating loop discovering an invaginated one. The latter is formed by an afferent (*1*) and an efferent segment (*2*). Suggestive and appropriate is the definition of invagination as a hernia of intestine into intestine. (*cont.* →)

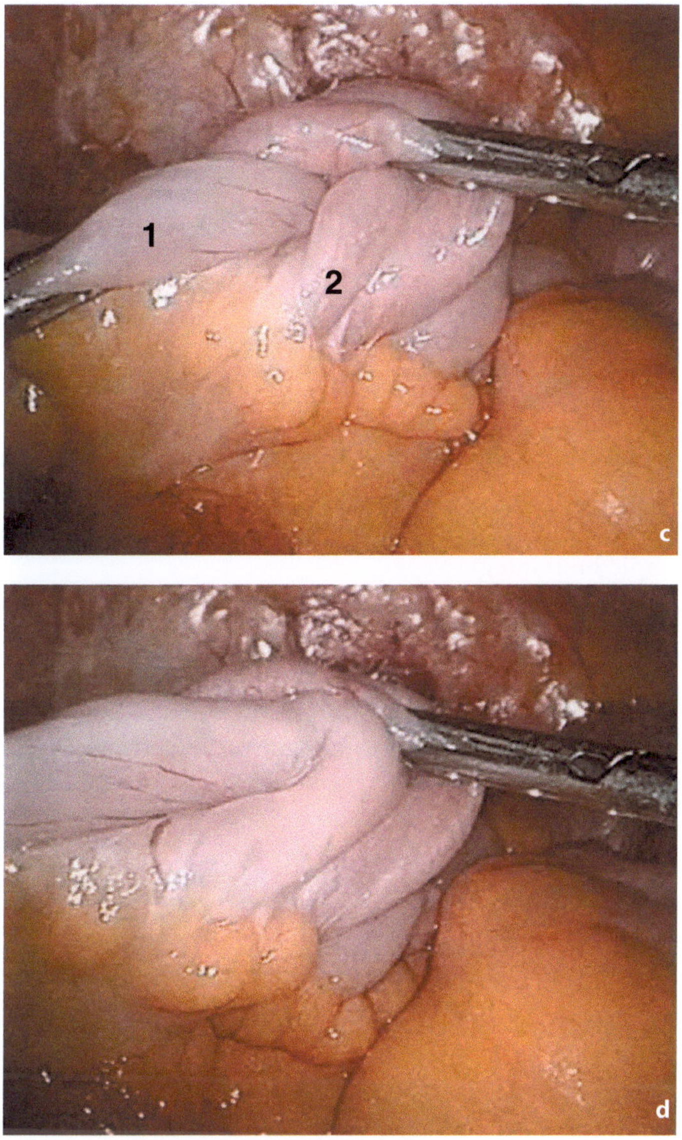

c The surgeon reduces invagination. *1* afferent loop, *2* efferent loop. **d** Invagination resolves, showing continuity of the afferent segment with the efferent one. Resection of about 7 cm of the small bowel, revealed the presence of a polyp, which created a wedge for intussusception

SBO by Large-Bowel Obstruction

Ileal–jejunal dilatation may be caused by an obstruction site localised in the colon. Contemporary presence of radiological findings involving both small and large bowel facilitates diagnosis. Stenotic alterations of the cecum/right colon may even produce acute intestinal appearances involving only the small bowel.

SBO by Intestinal Strangling and Strangulation

Intestinal strangling and strangulation cause problems of canalisation because of injury to the anatomofunctional loop mesentery complex. In this instance, vital effects of vascular and nervous impairment are added to those of canalisation interruption, which compromises organic and dynamic loop integrity.

In hernias, strangling acts as a compressive and concentric ring mechanism of the bowel and mesentery.

In volvulus, strangulation acts as an axial rotation mechanism of the bowel mesentery system (Fig. 1.7).

Clinically, these occlusions may produce rapid and dramatic changes, with progressive impairment of intestinal loops and their mesentery.

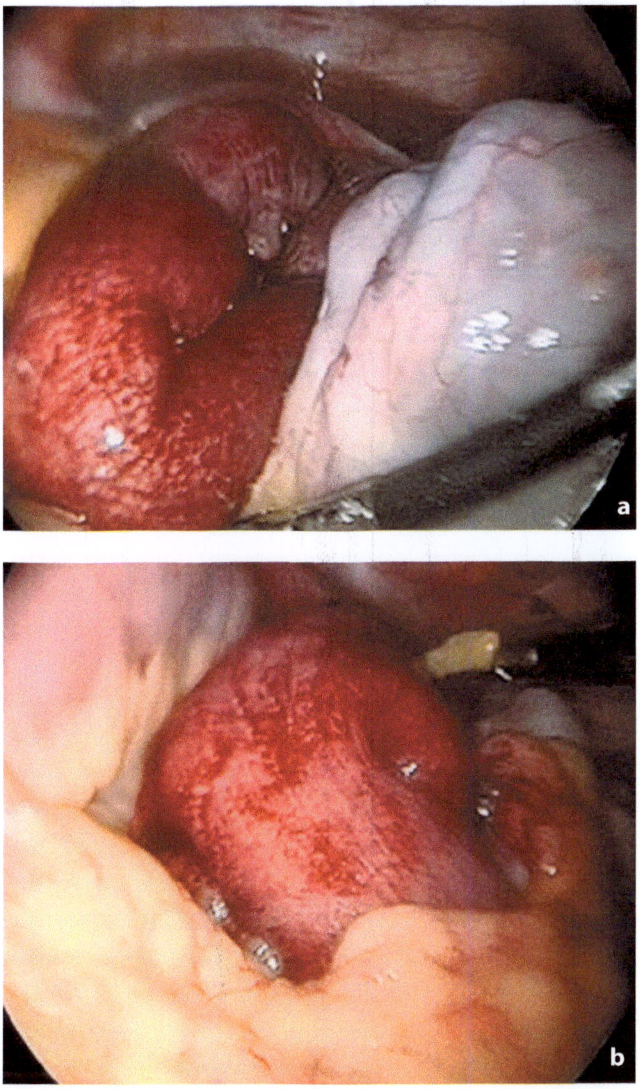

Fig. 1.7 a-f. Small-bowel obstruction by strangulation. Videolaparoscopic operation. Small-bowel volvulus due to adhesional band. **a, b** Small-bowel loops are seen from the free antimesenteric border with congested and thickened walls and haemorrhagic changes. (*cont.* →)

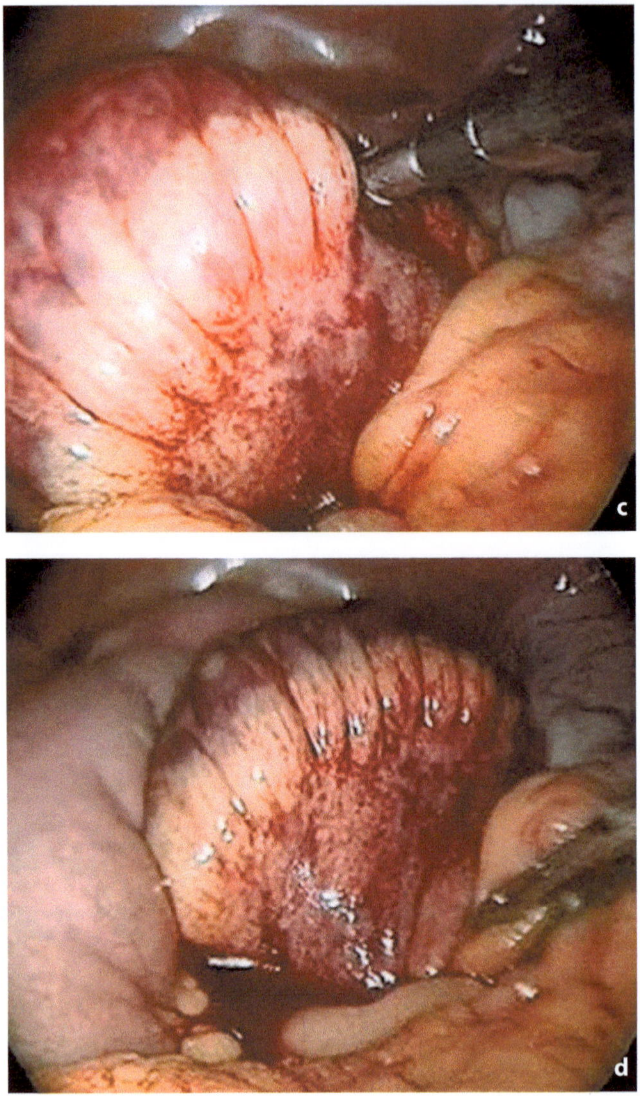

c, d Small-bowel volvulus with axial rotation of bowel–mesentery system. There is a thickened and haemorrhagic mesentery with blood-stained fluid in the peritoneal recesses of the mesentery. *(cont.* →)

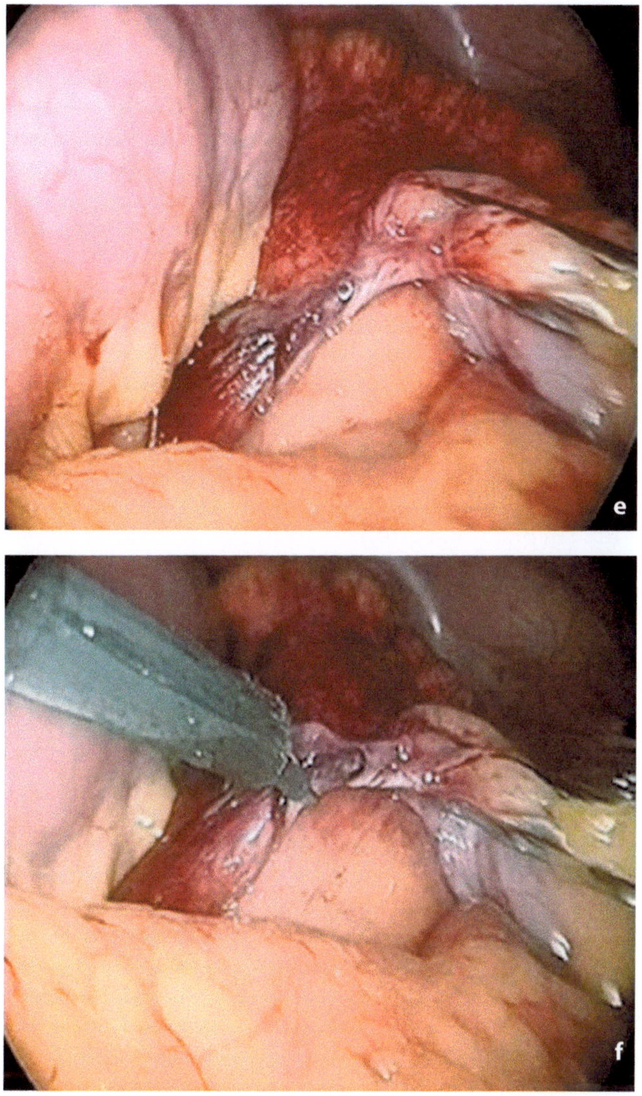

e, f Location of the band and adhesiolysis. Volvulus derotation, washings with tepid water and application of warm, damp patches allowed restoration of the bowel–mesentery complex

Complex Mechanisms

Complex mechanisms include a whole number of factors which, adding to the initial obstructive picture, modify it. They may change both configuration and extension of the obstructive pattern as well as its evolution.

The onset of complex mechanisms is unpredictable and multifactorial. For instance, tension and gravitational effects of the fluid-filled bowel loops may cause abnormal bowel angulation, torsion or volvulus.

To understand complex mechanisms of SBO, the following two cases are presented:

Case 1: An elderly patient quickly eats a huge quantity of cold corn meal mush. Corn meal mush creates an alimentary bolus, with SBO by obturation. The weight of the loops quickly creates a complex mechanism of serrated volvulus. Strangulation causes bowel necrosis, which necessitates wide surgical resection.

Case 2: A gastroresected patient eats 20 persimmons on a bet. This generates a phytobezoar that collects within a huge Meckel's diverticulum. The weighted diverticulum becomes the fulcrum of a segmentary ileal volvulus, but without strangulation (Fig. 1.8)

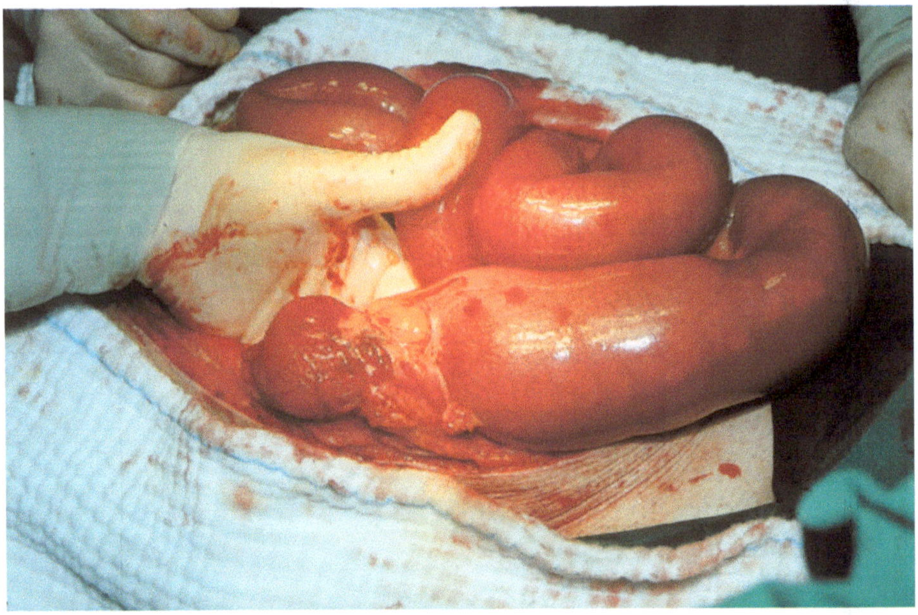

Fig. 1.8. Small-bowel obstruction by complex mechanism. A phytobezoar in large Meckel's diverticulum. The diverticulum, becomes heavier, and serves as a fulcrum to produce a segmentary small-bowel volvulus without strangulation. Meckel's diverticulum, significant bowel distension and abnormal location of bowel are visible. Walls are congested but not thickened

Volvulus

The term volvulus derives from the Latin verb *volvere* – to wrap up in coils – and defines loop torsion on its mesenteric axis: the mesentery wraps up in coils on itself. This mechanism causes abnormal location of loops and vessels, which appear converging towards the torsive point. Loops assume a spiral configuration. Vessels are stretched and twisted until the artery and vein are in an inverted position.

Volvulus may spontaneously resolve, and its formation does not necessarily imply strangulation of the feeding-vessel pedicle. The latter occurs only in cases of a particularly serrated strangulation.

Small-bowel volvulus should always be considered as secondary.

In our opinion, a complex mechanism is the cause of volvulus in Muslim patients during Ramadan: in such cases, after a long fast, a huge quantity of food rich in fibres is ingested. Thus, volvulus secondary to obturation obstruction by alimentary bolus may occur. Such volvulus has been improperly defined as primitive by some authors.

Closed Loop

Closed loop means an obstructed loop at two points along its course. Formation mechanism is sustained by a single obstructed focus, which interacts on two points of the same intestinal tract (Fig. 1.9).

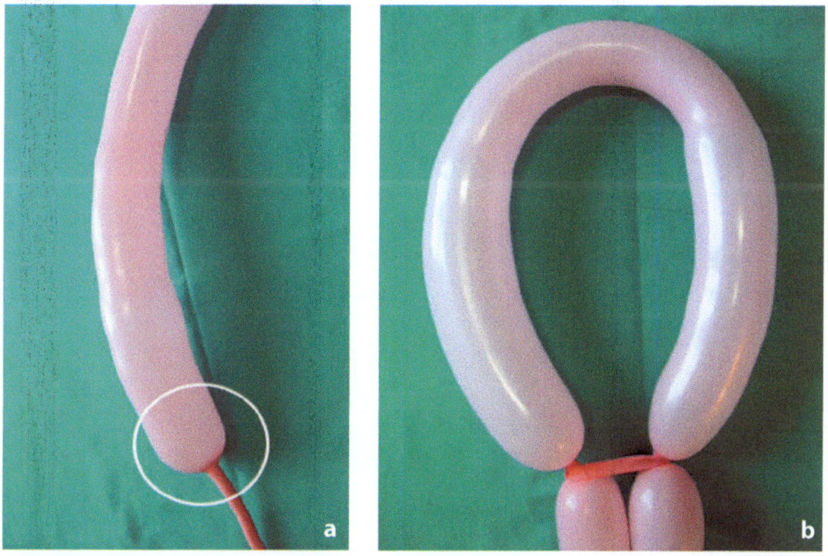

Fig. 1.9 a, b. a Simulation with a balloon of blockage obstruction due to adhesional band. Transition zone (*circle*) with the proximal part dilated and the distal part collapsed. **b** Simulation with a balloon of closed-loop obstruction due to adhesional band. Single obstructed focus interacts with two adjacent points of the arch of the balloon

Numerous formation mechanisms of SBO may generate a closed loop: it may be caused by an adhesional band, entrapped or incarcerated hernia or laparocele, or volvulus. It is important to stress that evidence of a closed loop is not synonymous with strangling or strangulation.

2 Computed Tomography Imaging Pathophysiology

R. Di Mizio, F. D'Amario, V. Di Mizio, M.A. Colasante, G. D'Amico, S. Altobelli, P. Innocenti, M. Scaglione

The main clinical and radiological problem consists of differentiating the obstruction with a purely occlusive risk from the obstruction in which vascular risk is added. The pure obstruction allows for elective surgery and a restoration of a more complete hydroelectrolytic equilibrium. Nasogastric intubation may avoid urgent surgical intervention. An additional benefit is that the tone and motility of the bowel loops and their intramural condition may improve with aspiration. The lower tension reduces stasis, intestinal diameter and intraperitoneal fluid, and it may sometimes completely resolve the occlusive condition. On the other hand, the obstruction with vascular risk does not show significant clinical improvement after nasogastric tube placement. Deliberation and delayed surgery must be avoided.

On the basis of surgical and imaging findings, we can differentiate small-bowel obstruction (SBO) as:

- simple;
- decompensated;
- complicated.

Simple SBO

The basis of SBO pathophysiology is distension of the bowel loops located proximally to the obstruction site. Increase in intraluminal tension distends the loop and forces reduction of tone, with a progressive increase of the diameter. Intestinal stasis is always of mixed variety: gaseous and liquid. The extreme intraluminal tension compresses and stretches the wall.

Intravenous (IV) contrast-enhanced computed tomography (CT) shows thin walls with preserved and homogeneous contrast enhancement (CE). Valvulae conniventes with an elegant complete circular design rapidly appear, indicating the extreme tone-kinetic attempt to exceed the mechanical occlusive obstacle. The crowded and forced attitude of the valvulae indicates functional shortening of the small bowel. This event is more significant in the jejunum, which – due to its nature – has a higher dynamic muscular efficacy. In effect, the jejunum is the true propulsive motor of the entire small bowel, and its activity in such case means hyperperistaltic motions.

In simple SBO, the vascular supply is preserved, and there is no peritoneal fluid. Nevertheless, the simple obstruction has an intrinsic evolutive dynamism.

Decompensated SBO

Usually, the gastrointestinal tract handles 8–9 l of fluid daily, most of which is reabsorbed by the small bowel. If the occlusive status persists, simple SBO develops into decompensated SBO. The increasing intraluminal tension causes a change of parietal microcirculation, which impairs bowel capability to reabsorb. This happens only when the intraluminal pressure is greater than the pressure into capillary vessels, causing an alteration of vascular permeability. The bowel loop progressively becomes decompensated. A definite flow of fluids forms outside the intestinal wall in the lumen and peritoneal cavity. Nevertheless, the wall does not become thicker, because the tension of the lumen squeezes it like a sponge. The stretched and squashed wall becomes thin and tight.

IV contrast-enhanced CT shows thin walls with preserved and homogeneous CE. The wall transudates fluid into and out of the loop. The fluid component of the intraluminal stasis increases, and it increasingly exceeds the gaseous component; the bowel, located distal to the occlusive focus, progressively collapses; a transudate appears in the peritoneal cavity. The intraperitoneal fluid will be initially found in the recesses between the loops, then in the peritoneal recesses of the mesentery and finally free in the peritoneal cavity. Surgery reveals the presence of peritoneal fluid with a cedar-like appearance.

As in all states of imbalance, the decompensated bowel may be acute or chronic, and it may resolve or deteriorate:

- **Acute decompensated bowel loop:** appears when the obstructive fulcrum suddenly acts and causes a sharp increase of intraluminal pressure.
- **Chronic decompensated bowel loop**: appears when the occlusion is inveterate.
- **Regression**: if the therapy reduces the tensive effect, the imbalance regresses, with a progressive reduction of loop diameter, of liquid stasis, and of intraperitoneal fluid.
- **Deterioration**: if the dilatation persists, the occlusion worsens. Repeatedly, the tension causes a reduction in arterial blood flow with a progressive impoverishment of intramural perfusion, which contributes to the increasingly thinner appearance of the walls. IV contrast-enhanced

CT shows thin walls with preserved and homogeneous CE. Surgery reveals distended and pale loops.

The decompensated bowel repeatedly causes a peritoneal reaction due to involvement of the visceral serosa. Surgery reveals the presence of more or less turbid peritoneal liquid.

In the event of unsuccessful treatment, the natural evolution of the SBO is towards death by consumption. The parietal ischaemic deficit joins the progressive drop in neuromuscular tone. The loops become increasingly dilated with very thin walls – like Egyptian papyrus – without tone, motility or elasticity. The terminal picture is that of intestinal digestive secretion impairment. The SBO becomes an adynamic paralytic ileus.

The inveterate ischaemia causes trophic mural changes, which predispose to progressive erosion ⟹ fissuration ⟹ laceration ⟹ diastasic perforation and ultimately peritonitis. Perforation of the wall is due to the mechanical effect of loop distension. The phenomena of atrophy and necrosis are more evident on the antimesenteric border of the loop.

In both simple and decompensated SBO, the mortality rate is approximately 3%.

Complicated SBO

Complicated SBO means an occlusive state complicated by vascular changes of the bowel wall. These complications may present with two different modalities:

- vascular changes due to strangling and strangulation (Fig. 2.1);
- vascular changes due to fight (Fig. 2.2).

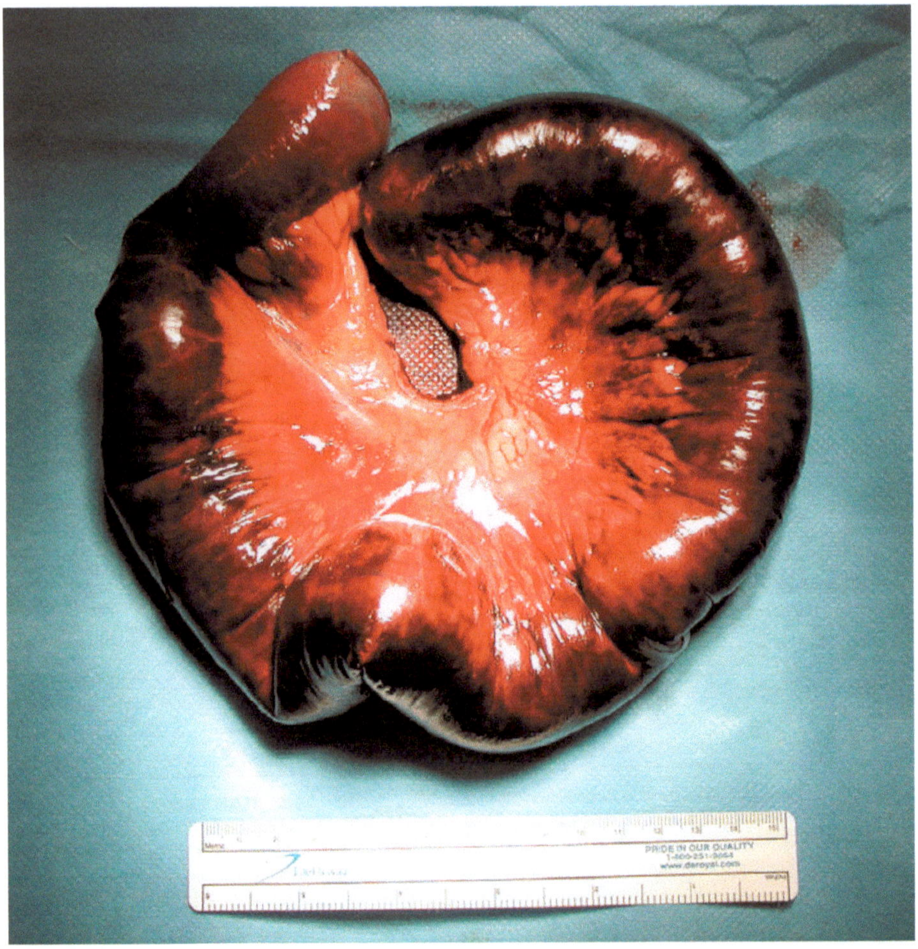

Fig. 2.1. Vascular changes due to strangulation. Intestinal necrotic segment due to strangulated volvulus by adhesional band. Thickened loop, with a spotted dark red or frankly anthracite black colour. Diffuse haemorrhage of the mesentery

Vascular Changes due to Strangling and Strangulation

The mechanisms of strangling and strangulation involve the loop and its mesentery. In these cases, the perfusion deficit involves the venous circulation, which is easily compressible and collapsible. Impairment of arterial circulation occurs very late. The obstacle to the blood outflow causes:

- Intramural venous congestion with pathological wall thickening of the loop. Surgery reveals the presence of congested loops with haemorrhage, with a colour varying from dark red – like wine dregs – to black anthracite. IV contrast-enhanced CT shows thickened walls with altered CE.
- Haemorrhagic engorgement of the mesentery: the swollen and oedematous mesentery curves the loops anteriorly, spacing them out. There is prominent vasculature with numerous dilated vessels.

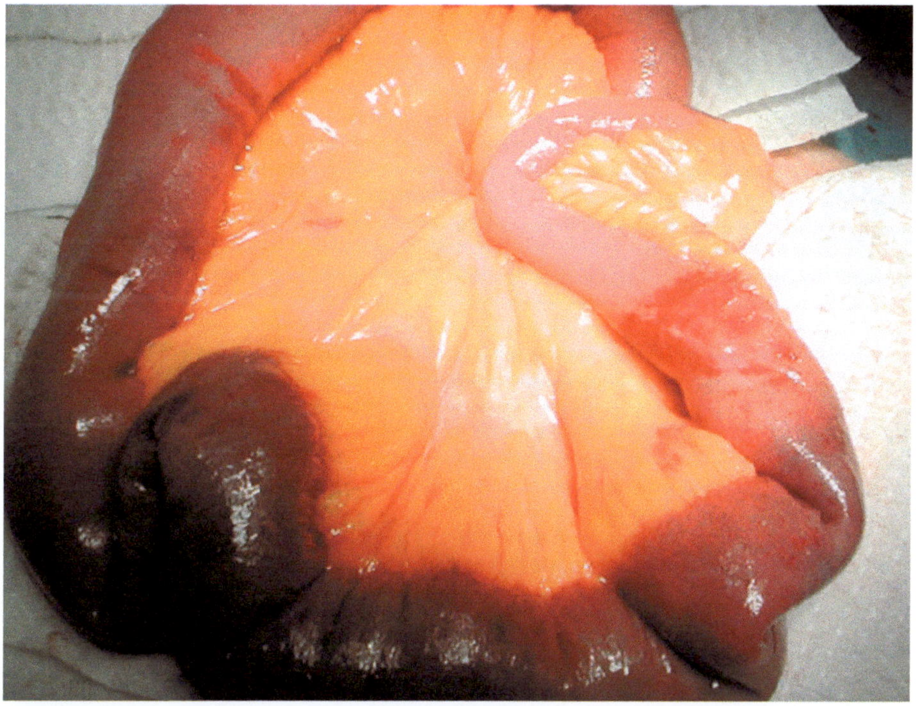

Fig. 2.2. Vascular changes due to fight. Crural hernia with incarceration of ileal loops, which appear distended and thickened, with haemorrhagic effusion. Mesentery is preserved. Surgeon has performed washings with tepid water and has applied warm damp patches for several minutes. Loops have recovered their vitality

- Early appearance of peritoneal fluid: the intraperitoneal fluid will be initially found in the recesses between the loops, then in mesenteric recesses and finally free in the peritoneal cavity. Surgery reveals the presence of serohaemorrhagic or merely haemorrhagic fluid. The percentage of blood in the peritoneal fluid influences its tomodensitometric values.

Strangulation has been observed in 10–15% of patients who underwent surgery for SBO. Frager DH et al. (see "Selected Readings") report a mortality of about 8% if surgical intervention is performed within 36 h from symptom onset. After 36 h, mortality increases to about 25%.

Vascular Changes due to Fight

In the evolution of SBO, vascular suffering due to fight may appear. Vascular changes due to fight have a district location and appear only when the intramural venous circulation significantly slows down. The origin of this event is multifactorial and unpredictable. The main factors are:

- the obstructive mechanism, occlusion duration and onset of complex mechanisms;
- the mesenteric and enteric circulation, already uncertain due to diffuse atherosclerotic disease;
- the pathological remains, which alter the abdominal habitat;
- the patient's age and general status.

IV contrast-enhanced CT shows high CE in the wall, with normal or borderline thickness. The continuous vascular afflux causes repeated engorgement and vascular dilatation with intramural congestion: the wall becomes thick. IV contrast-enhanced CT shows homogeneous high CE in a thick wall without stratification. The parietal changes initially involve the mesenteric border.

Sometimes, mild involvement of mesenteric circulation may be present, with slowing and stasis. Actually, minimal alterations of the vascular bed and mesenteric fat may appear, exclusively located at the mesenteric–intestinal junction.

Usually, a loop due to fight is near the obstructive site. The venous congestion of the loop may cause passage of blood into the peritoneal cavity. Surgery may reveal serohaemorrhagic fluid. Definitively, the fight obstruction causes change wall density and thickness. Mesenteric involvement is absent or minimal.

Common Aspects of Loop Vascular Changes

Regardless of the cause, in the initial phase, the loop vascular change are a reversible phenomenon, with the possible recovery of intestinal vitality and function. During surgery, the specialist performs washings with tepid water and applies warm, damp patches for several minutes. Vitality restoration is evident by the reappearance of peristalsis and the progressive recovery of colour.

Without a timely resolution, the natural history of this acute secondary venous ischemia is progression to necrosis ⟹ gangrene ⟹ perforation ⟹ peritonitis.

Intramural haemorrhage is typically accompanied by severe inflammation, with further wall damage. The intestinal stasis favours the intraluminal growth of microbes. If the mucosal barrier is interrupted, the loop undergoes bacterial invasion. The parietal perfusion changes favour the growth of germ cultures, with intramural infection. Moreover, interruption of the mucosal barrier allows the passage of gas from the intestinal lumen into the wall, thence into the mesenteric venous system, and finally into the portal venous system.

Repeatedly, this progressive and worsening venous engorgement of the mesentery is followed by a reflex arterial spasm, either local or diffuse. The blood is deflected towards other vital organs. The amount of IV contrast that arrives at the loop wall is dramatically reduced: CE will be poor or absent.

Intramural necrosis causes inflammation of the visceral serosa. Usually, the diffuse peritoneal complications appear slowly. Nevertheless, their early appearance may be prompted by rapid worsening of the pathologic condition, which frequently occurs in elderly patients. The SBO develops into a peritonitic paralytic ileus.

3 Computed Tomography Features

R. Di Mizio, F. D'Amario, V. Di Mizio, A. Filippone, L. Romano, M. Scaglione

The development in helical computed tomography (CT) from single-detector to multidetector equipment has overcome peristaltic intestinal artefacts, allowing optimal bowel visualisation and contrast enhancement (CE). As a result, this permits a finer representation and a more accurate evaluation of the bowel and mesentery. Furthermore, technological advances now allow optimal multiplanar reconstruction (MPR). To date, contrast-enhanced multidetector CT (MDCT) has become the gold standard in the evaluation of small-bowel obstruction (SBO).

Examination Technique

In suspected SBO, MDCT can be used both as first imaging modality and for integrative study. For obvious radiation-dose-related issues, the CT technique varies in these two situations:
CT as first-imaging modality: includes scout views (frontal and lateral) and a scan before and after intravenous (IV) contrast material
CT for integrative study: includes a frontal scout view and a scan after IV contrast material

In our practice, in patients with SBO, MDCT is not performed with oral and/or rectal contrast agents. The study of the bowel walls requires tailored injection of an IV iodinated contrast agent.
130 ml of IV contrast agent at the concentration of 400 mg iodine/millilitre (ml) (Iomeron 400, Bracco, Italy) are continuously injected in the following way: the first bolus of 50 ml is injected at the rate of 1.5 ml/s, followed by a second bolus of 80 ml at the rate of 3 ml/s. The scan delay is 70 s. This protocol allows simultaneous, optimal enhancement of the arteries and the mucosa (provided by the second bolus) and, in the same way, the slighter depiction of the veins and the bowel wall (supported by the first bolus). As a result, the abdomen "lights up" for simultaneous enhancement of the bowel wall, the vessels and the parenchyma, allowing the possibility of analysing all abdominal and intestinal component with significant radia-

tion-dose reduction. MPR is very helpful in analysing such a complex and convoluted structure as the small bowel. In fact, MPR may be very useful in correctly interpreting equivocal findings on axial scans. The overall accuracy of diagnostic confidence is significantly higher when axial scans are assessed with MPR simultaneously.

CT Findings

CT findings are presented according to the CT report. At contrast-enhanced CT:

- Simple SBO is characterised by evaluation of the bowel.
- In decompensated SBO, the bowel and peritoneal cavity are depicted.
- Complicated SBO due to strangling and strangulation is characterised by depiction of a thickened bowel and mesentery.
- Complicated SBO due to fight is characterised by depiction of a thickened bowel. Vascular changes due to fight have a focal location and appear only when the intramural venous circulation significantly slows down.

Simple SBO

Bowel Images (Figs. 3.1–3.6)

According to the literature, the jejunum and the ileum are considered thickened if their diameter increases above 3 cm and 2.5 cm, respectively. The thickness of the wall of a dilated loop is considered pathologic if it exceeds 2 mm:

- Dilated loops proximal to the transition zone.
- Transition zone (point of obstruction) is defined as the abrupt diameter change between the dilated and the collapsed loops. Its shape depends on the cause, the mechanism of obstruction and the scan plane. Identification of the transition zone is not always possible. The typical "bird-beak" appearance, described in the literature, is sometimes demonstrable. At other times – for instance, in obstruction caused by an alimentary bolus – the transition zone presents as a heterogeneous intraluminal mass without CE.
- Collapsed loops distal to the point of obstruction.
- Mixed enteric stasis, gaseous and liquid. A faecaloid enteric stasis, defined in the literature as the "small-bowel faeces sign", is sometimes visible. The pathogenesis of this sign is multifactorial: for instance, slow intestinal transit, enteric secretion and absorption abnormalities, or place-

ment of a nasogastric tube. The faecal material may invade the distal ileum when the ileocecal valve is incompetent. The small-bowel faeces sign is a nonspecific finding of SBO, detectable also on plain film and ultrasonography (US).

- Normal and thin walls with homogeneous and regular CE.
- At the jejunum, the presence of multiple, crowded, thin valvulae conniventes equal to one another.
- Scantly detectable or collapsed colic frame; preserved and homogeneous colon CE.
- Normal and transparent mesentery.
- Normal and preserved mesenteric vascularity.
- Absence of peritoneal fluid.

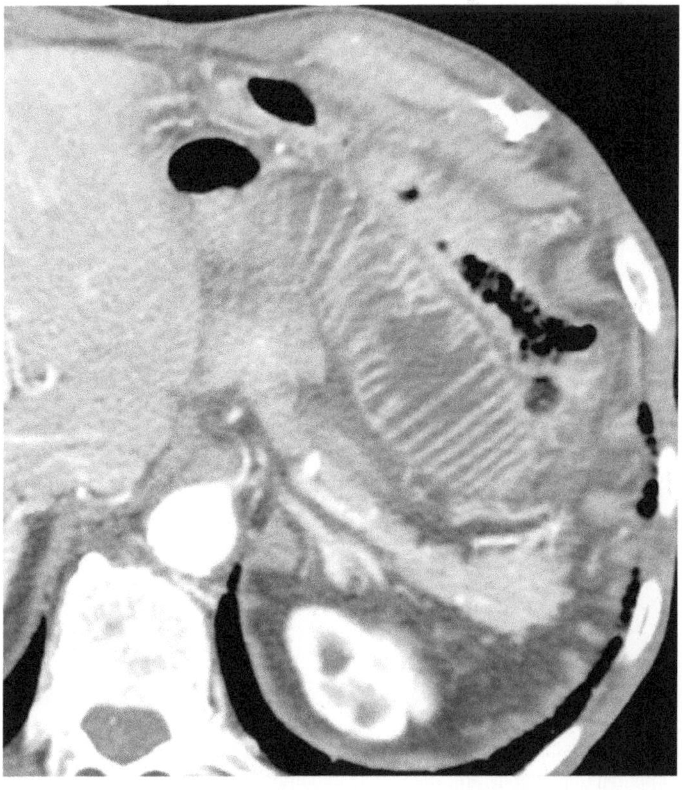

Fig. 3.1. Simple small-bowel obstruction. Contrast-enhanced multidetector computed tomography. In the left upper abdomen, a fluid-filled, dilated jejunal loop is evident. The bowel walls are normal and thin with typical contrast enhancement. The valvulae conniventes are numerous, crowded and thin. The packed and forced appearance of the valvulae conniventes is related to the functional reduction of the small bowel, which acts like a spring in an extreme tone-kinetic attempt to overcome the obstructive obstacle

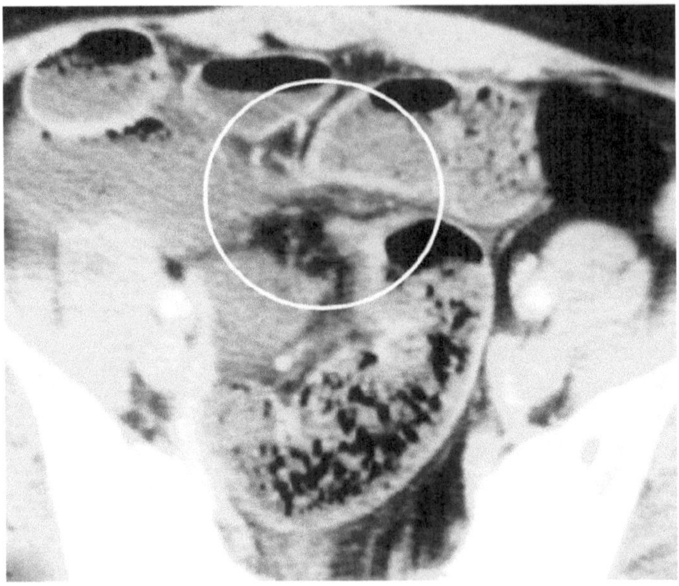

Fig. 3.2. Simple small-bowel obstruction due to adhesional band. Contrast-enhanced multidetector computed tomography. At the transition point, a dilated loop with typical "bird-beak" aspect (*circle*). Proximal to the transition point, dilated loops with faecal-like content. The bowel walls are normal with normal contrast enhancement

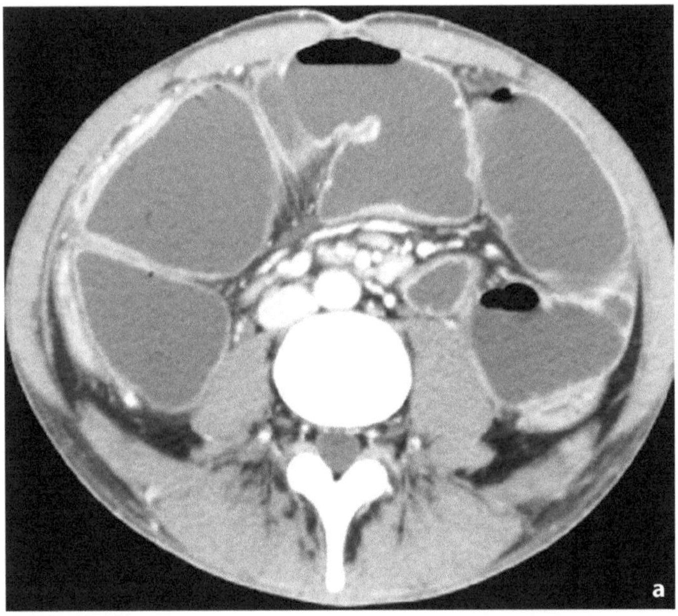

Fig. 3.3 a-c. Simple small-bowel obstruction due to Crohn's enteritis. Contrast-enhanced multidetector computed tomography. **a** In the middle abdomen, dilated small-bowel loops mainly fluid filled. Normal and thin bowel walls with typical contrast enhancement. The mesentery is normal. Regular vascularity. Simultaneous enhancement of the arterial and venous system allows optimal identification of the multiple lymphadenopathies. (*cont.* →)

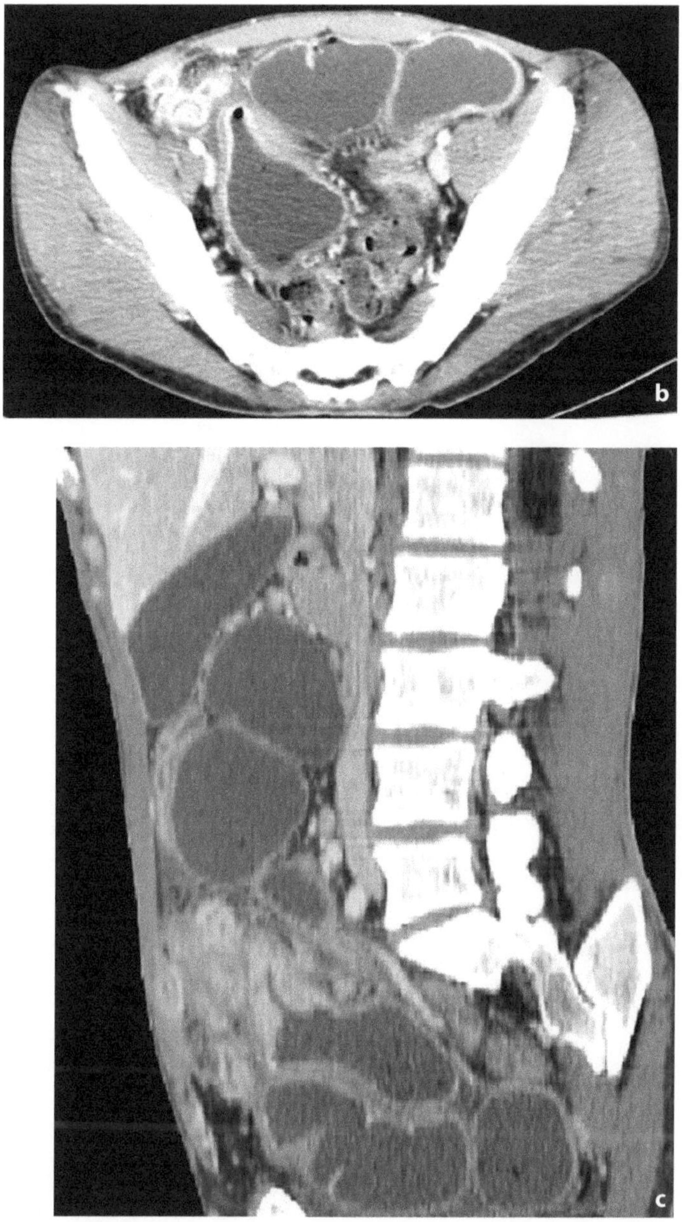

b At the pelvic level, a funnel-shaped, serrated stenosis of the bowel lumen is evident, with dilated loops proximal to the obstruction site. Collapsed loops distal to the obstruction site. Crohn's disease causes by marked parietal thickness, mainly fibrotic. Absence of free fluid in the peritoneal cavity. **c** Parasagittal multiplanar reconstruction shows filiform-shaped lumen. The bowel wall is thick and fibrotic. Surgical resolution of mechanical obstruction by narrowing the lumen

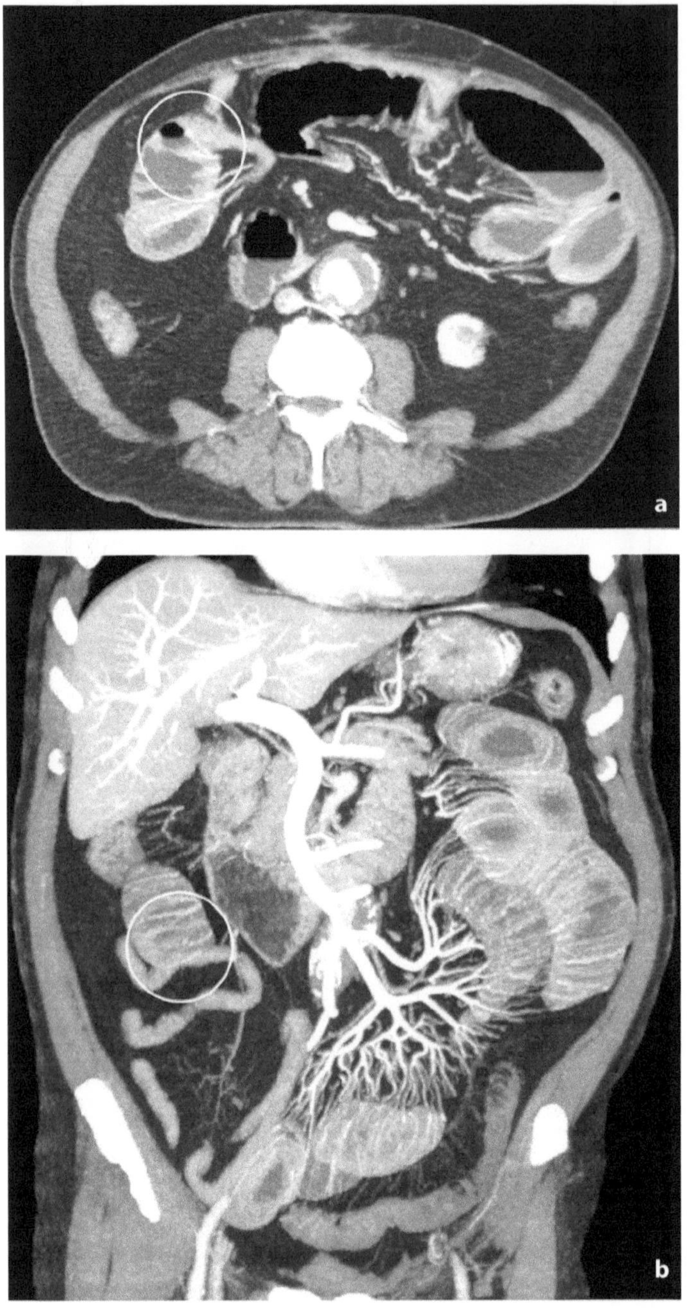

Fig. 3.4 a, b. Simple small-bowel obstruction due to adhesional band. Contrast-enhanced multidetector computed tomography. **a** Axial scan. **b** Combined multiplanar reconstruction and maximum intensity projection on oblique coronal plane. Dilated jejunal loops proximal to the transition zone (*circle*), easily detectable by the sudden diameter change. Collapsed loops distal to the point of obstruction. Normal bowel walls with thin valvulae conniventes and homogeneous contrast enhancement. The mesentery is normotransparent. Normal mesenteric vascularity. Absence of fluid in the peritoneal cavity. Dilated, calcified, thrombotic aorta

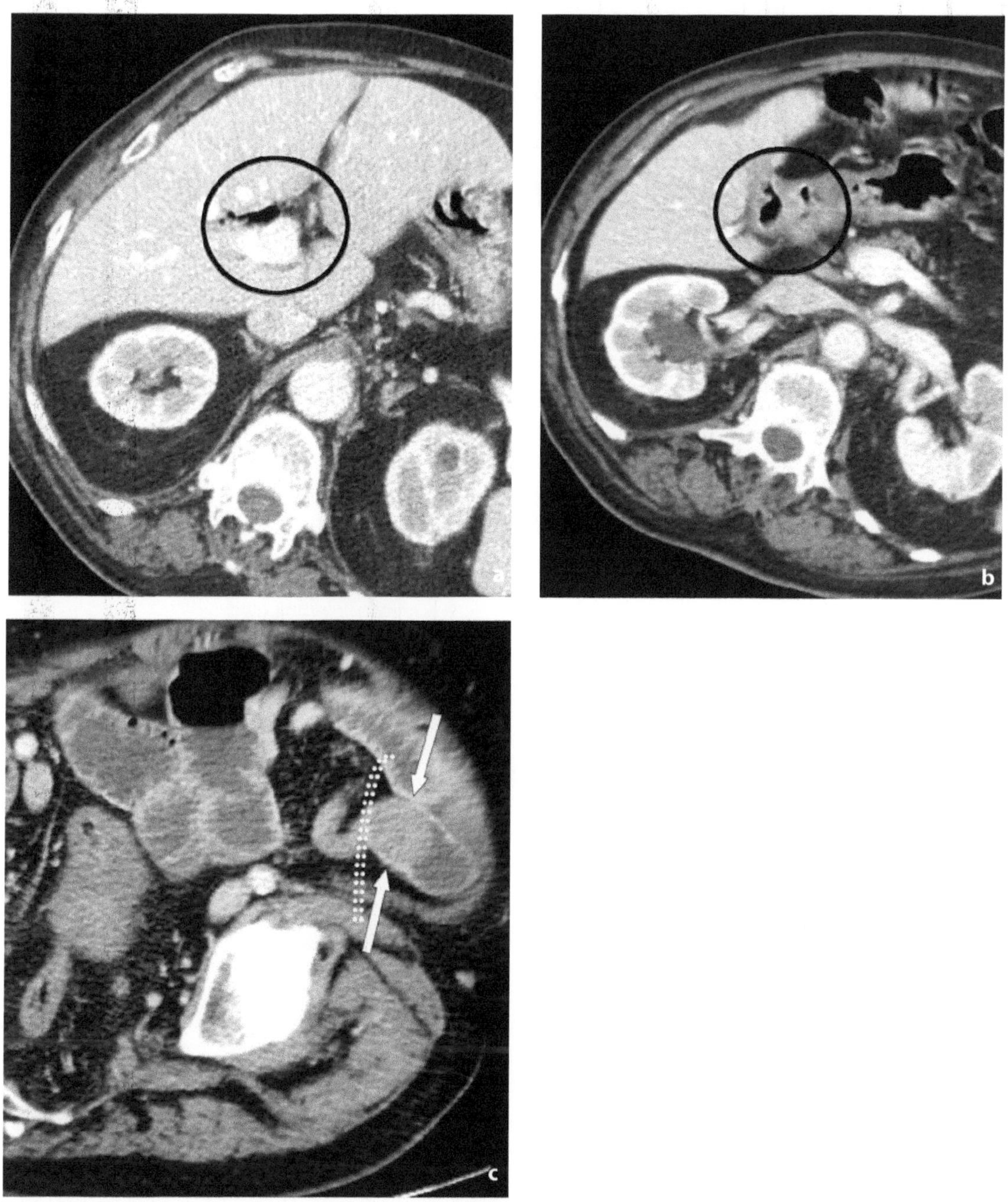

Fig. 3.5 a-c. Simple small-bowel obstruction (SBO). Contrast-enhanced multidetector computed tomography (CT). At the level of the liver, CT scans show air in the biliary tree (**a**) and gallbladder fistula (**b**). **c** CT scan of the mid-abdomen. There are dilated jejunal loops with mixed stasis. Thin bowel walls with normal contrast enhancement. At the level of the transition zone (*small dots*), a soft, radiopaque biliary stone (*arrows*) is evident. The mesentery is normal. Absence of fluid in the peritoneal cavity. Surgery revealed that the biliary stone impacted in a small-bowel loop, with abnormal angulation, depending on perivisceral chronic adhesional phenomenon. The obturation of the lumen due to a biliary stone as well as impairment due to the adhesional band determined the complex mechanism of SBO formation

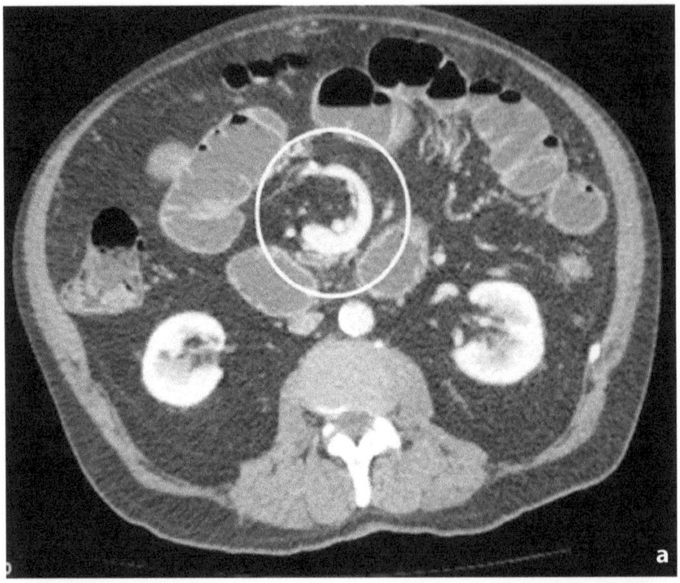

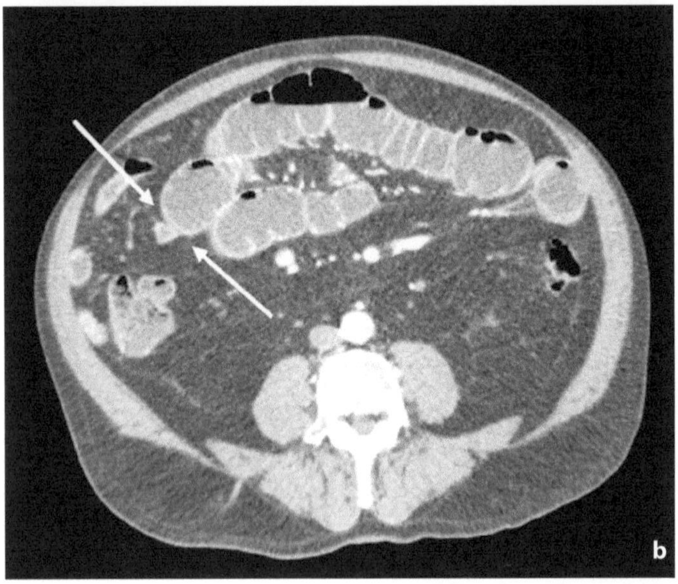

Fig. 3.6 a–d. Simple small-bowel obstruction by volvulus secondary to adhesional band. **a** Axial scan. Whirl sign, suggesting a mesenteric rotation upon itself (*circle*). Dilated small-bowel loops with mixed stasis. Thin bowel walls with normal contrast enhancement. **b** Axial scan. **c** Coronal multiplanar reconstruction (MPR). **d** Parasagittal MPR. *Arrows* and *circles* identify the transition zone with sudden small-bowel diameter change. Likely diagnosis of adhesional band. The mesentery and mesenteric vascularity appear normal. Absence of fluid in the peritoneal cavity. Distended gallbladder (*cont.* →)

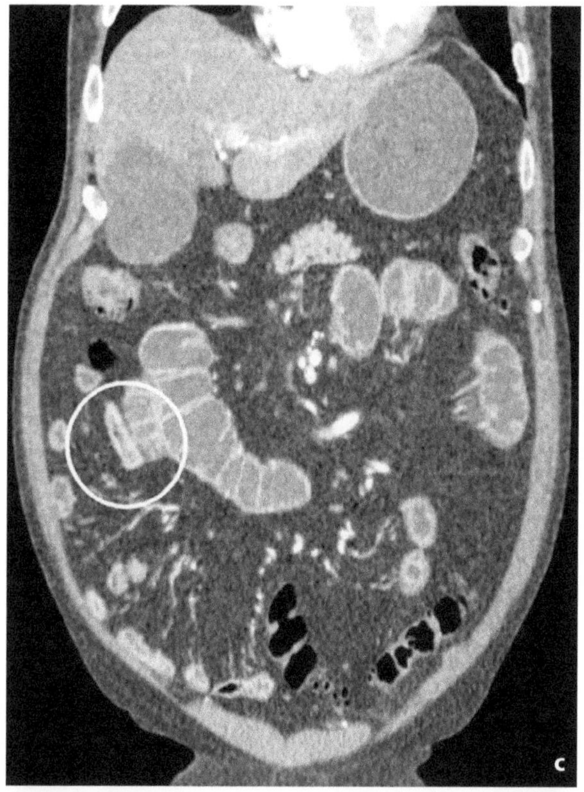

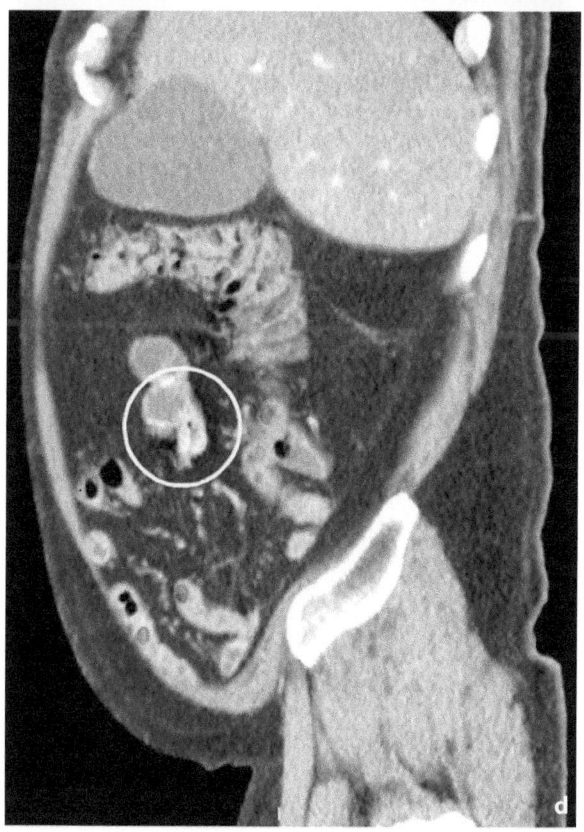

Decompensated SBO

Bowel and Peritoneal Cavity Images (Figs. 3.7–3.15)

CT of decompensated SBO consists of the bowel image of simple SBO in addition to findings related to the peritoneal cavity:

- Dilated loops with normal and thin walls with homogeneous CE, whose density may progressively decrease with vascular compromise.
- Mixed enteric stasis; usually, it is mainly liquid.
- Normal and transparent mesentery.
- Normal and preserved mesenteric vascularity.
- Extraluminal fluid between the dilated loops; this fluid shows typical triangular configuration reminiscent of a particular modern swimsuit – the tanga – and is thus often referred to as the "tanga sign".
- Fluid in the peritoneal recesses of the mesentery.
- Free fluid in the peritoneal cavity.

Follow-up

Simple and decompensated SBO may resolve after medical therapy and placement of a nasogastric tube and can be easily assessed and followed-up with serial plain films eventually integrated with US.

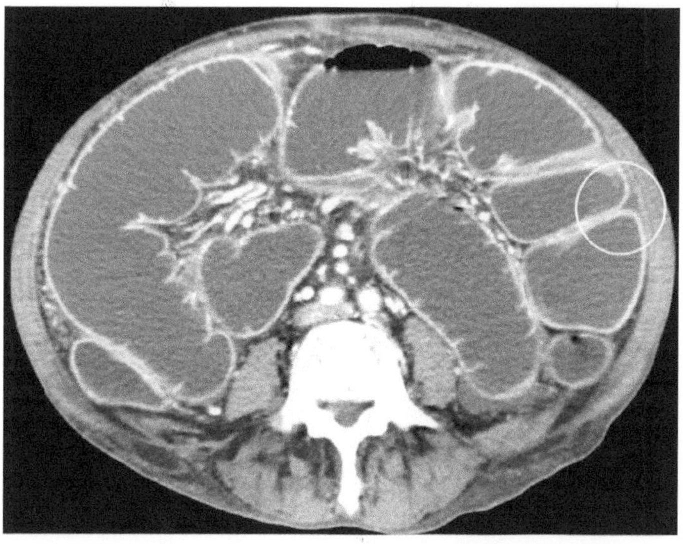

Fig. 3.7. Decompensated small-bowel obstruction. Contrast-enhanced multidetector computed tomography. Dilated small-bowel loops with thin walls and normal contrast enhancement. The mesentery is normal. Typical vascularity. *Circle* identifies a small amount of free fluid in the typical triangular configuration (tanga sign) in the recesses between the bowel loops. Fluid in the peritoneal cavity

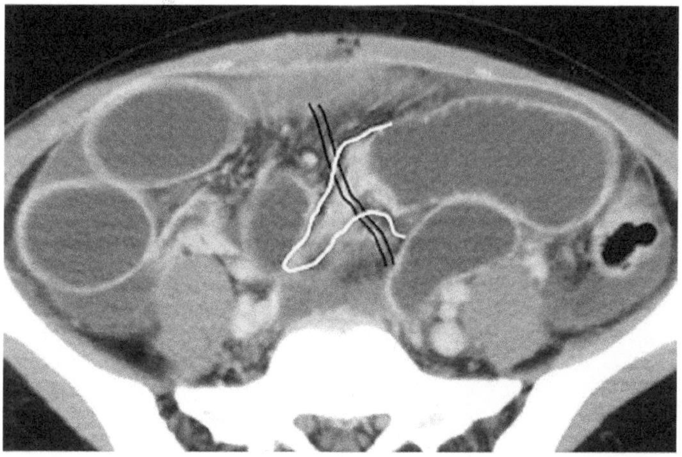

Fig. 3.8. Decompensated small-bowel obstruction. Contrast-enhanced multidetector computed tomography. Dilated small-bowel loops proximal to the transition zone – the "bird-beak" sign (*white line*) – secondary to blockage by adhesional band (*black lines*). Thin bowel walls and normal contrast enhancement. Normal mesentery

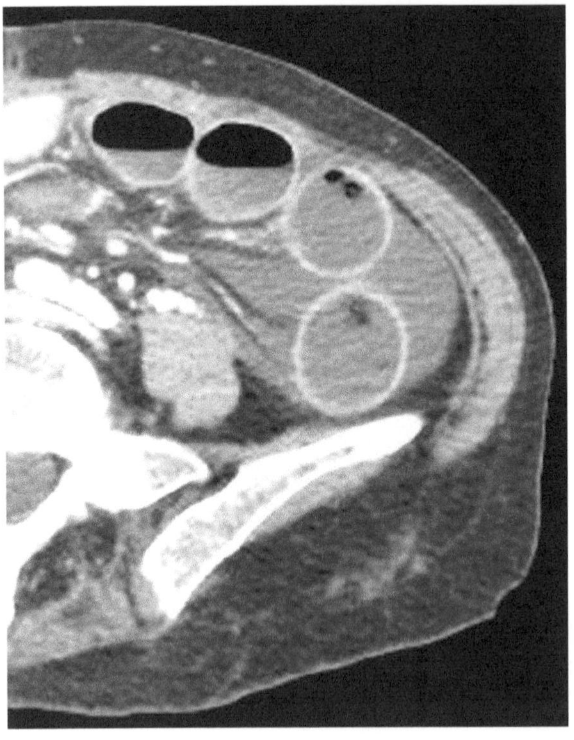

Fig. 3.9. Decompensated small-bowel obstruction. Contrast-enhanced multidetector computed tomography. Bowel and peritoneal cavity images. Dilated loops with normal walls. Mixed enteric stasis, gaseous and liquid. Free fluid in the peritoneal cavity and in the recesses of the mesentery. The mesenteric vessels and their adipose sheet are normotransparent

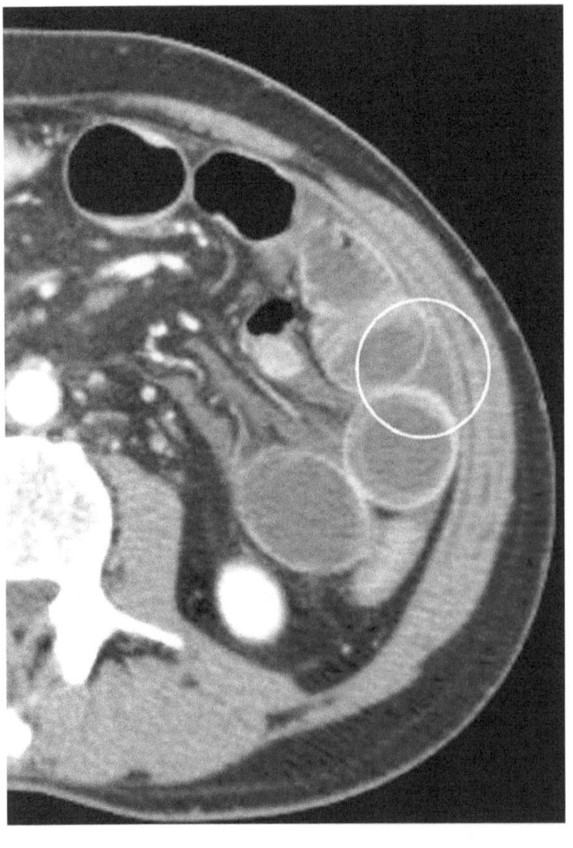

Fig. 3.10. Decompensated small-bowel obstruction. Contrast-enhanced multidetector computed tomography. Bowel and peritoneal cavity images. Fluid in the typical triangular configuration (tanga sign) (*circle*). The free fluid in the peritoneal recesses of the mesentery has a tendency to pool. This feature should not be misinterpreted as mesenteric vascular compromise. Actually, the adipose sheet of the mesenteric vessels is intact

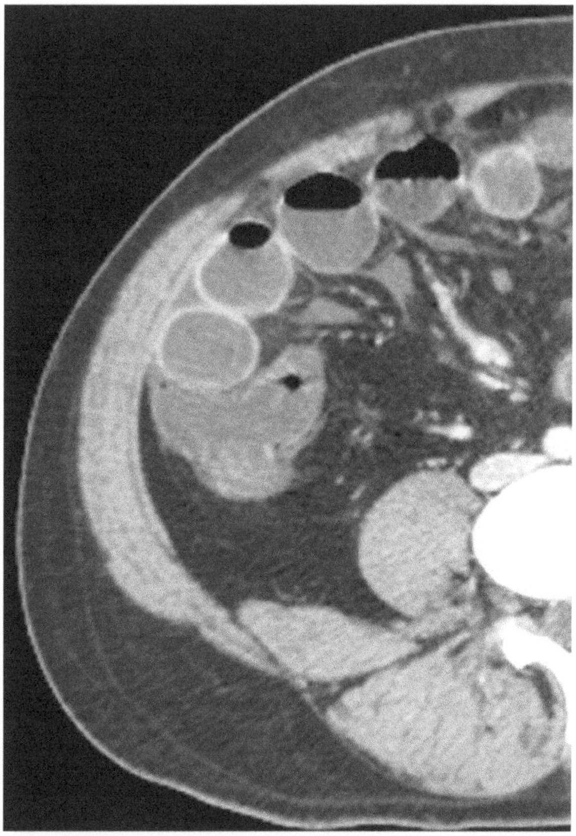

Fig. 3.11. Decompensated small-bowel obstruction. Contrast-enhanced multidetector computed tomography. Images of bowel and peritoneal cavity. At the mesenteric recesses, free fluid may take on bizarre shapes. The adipose sheet of the mesenteric vessels is normotransparent

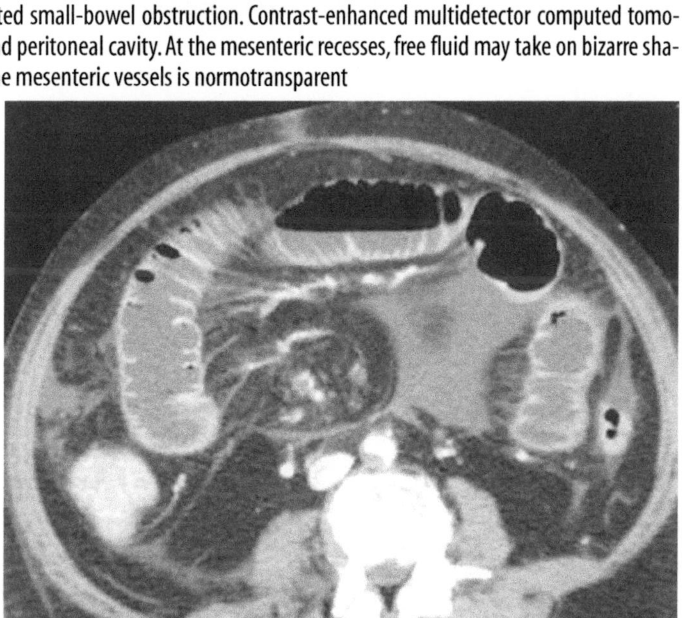

Fig. 3.12. Decompensated small-bowel obstruction. Contrast-enhanced multidetector computed tomography. Dilated small-bowel loops with thin walls, normal contrast enhancement and liquid–gaseous stasis. Collapsed colon. Abundant amount of fluid, particularly in the mesenteric recesses. The mesentery and vessels are intact

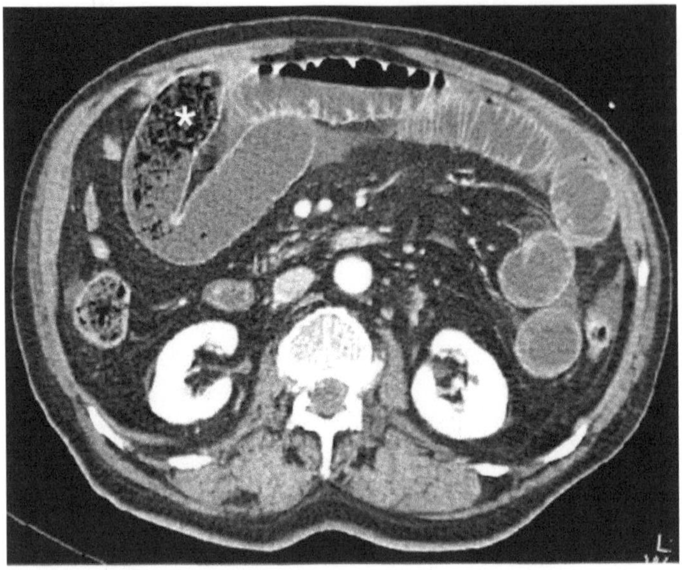

Fig. 3.13. Decompensated small-bowel obstruction. Contrast-enhanced multidetector computed tomography. At the level of the transition zone, a noncontrast, inhomogeneous, intraluminal mass (*asterisk*) due to phytobezoar is evident. Dilated bowel loops with thin walls and normal contrast enhancement. Mainly liquid stasis. Colonic frame scantly represented. The mesentery is normal. Small amount of free fluid in the peritoneal cavity

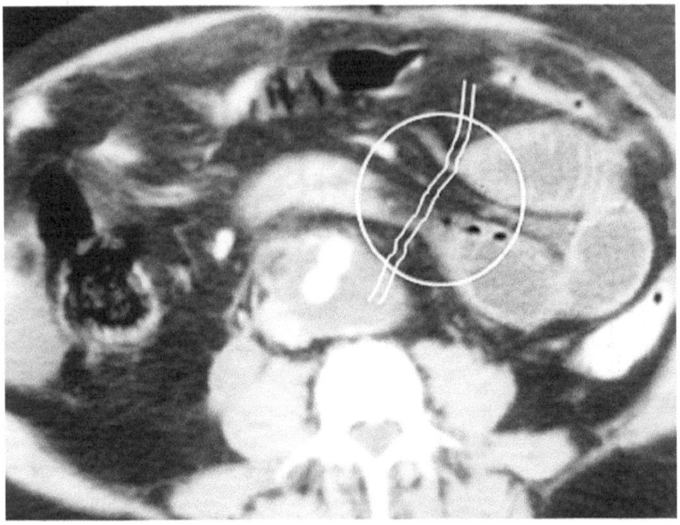

Fig. 3.14. Decompensated small-bowel obstruction. Contrast-enhanced multidetector computed tomography. Blockage due to adhesional band (*white lines*) acts on the adjacent points of a jejunal loop (*circle*), forming a closed loop. Thin bowel walls and normal contrast enhancement. Free focal peritoneal fluid in the mesenteric recess. Dilated, calcified, thrombotic aorta

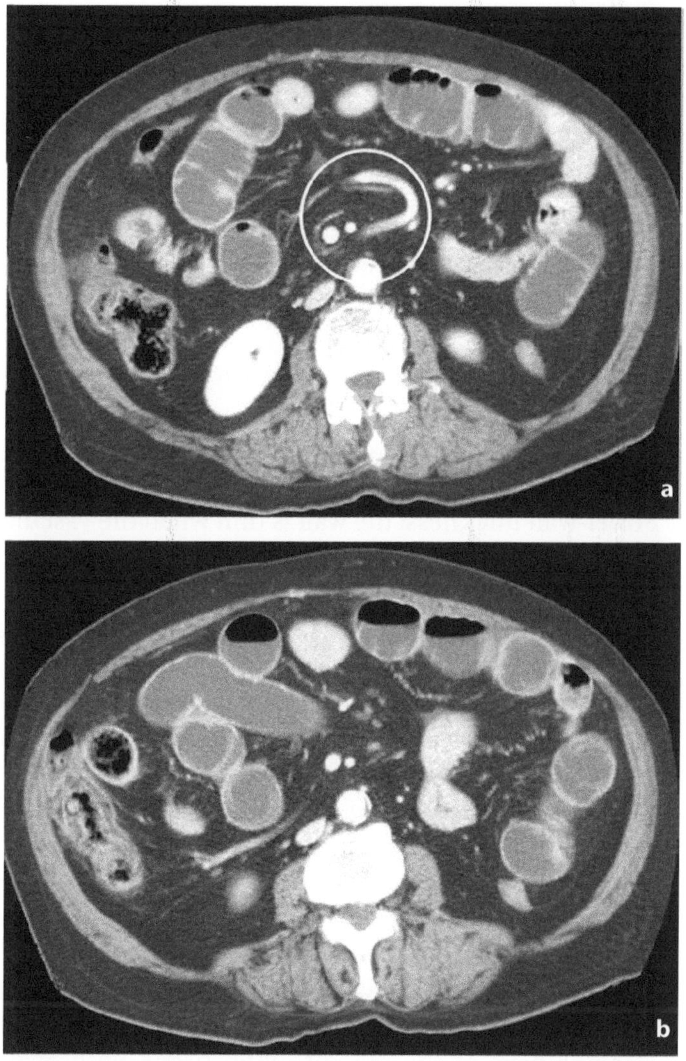

Fig. 3.15 a, b. Decompensated small-bowel obstruction by ileal volvulus due to adhesional band. Contrast-enhanced multidetector computed tomography. Twisted mesenteric vessels: whirl sign (*circle*). Dilated small bowel with mainly liquid content and preserved wall. The dilated loops are intervalled with contracted "white" loops due to hyperperistalsis. Small amount of fluid in the peritoneal cavity

Complicated SBO due to Strangling and Strangulation

Thickened Bowel and Mesentery Images (Figs. 3.16–3.26)

Strangling and strangulation of the small intestine are characterised by thickened bowel wall and vascular changes, with significant involvement of the mesentery and the peritoneal cavity. Imaging usually documents a clear clinical situation:

- Dilated loops proximal to the transition zone.
- Transition zone.
- Collapsed loops distal to the point of obstruction.
- Mixed enteric stasis with marked prevalence of liquid stasis.
- Bowel-wall thickness: the wall is thin when the vascular supply is normal; in cases of vascular compromise, there is circumferential wall thickening.
- Bowel-wall abnormality on CE: after contrast agent injection, the intestinal wall with vascular changes may present different patterns according to the severity of the vascular injury. The spectrum of CT features ranges from thickened bowel wall with high CE to total absence of CE. Between these two extreme conditions, numerous and different patterns may occur. They differ for presence or absence of mural stratification, variability in CE, entity of bowel thickness, and degree of bowel distension. Different patterns may occur simultaneously. The absence of or inadequate CE indicates arterial reflex spasm, as a consequence of bowel-injury severity. At present, pathophysiological features corresponding to the bowel-injury patterns have not been conclusively established.
- The thickened loop becomes rigid and loses its morphology.
- Wall pneumatosis with lamellar shape or intramural gas bubbles.
- Haemorrhage of the mesentery fat tissue, with hazy, opaque, mist and thickening; loss of transparency of the fat sheet around the mesenteric vessels. These findings may be focal, confined to the obstruction site, or diffuse, involving a wide portion of the mesentery. Sometimes, mesenteric haziness may appear before the CT finding of pathologic bowel thickening.
- Congestion and engorgement of the mesenteric vessels with prominent vasculature. To correctly evaluate the status of the mesenteric vasculature, biological comparison to normal vessels is crucial. The arterial reflex spasm, diffuse or focal, occurs later and determines the reduction in diameter and number of vessels.
- Gas in the superior mesenteric vein.
- Gas in the portal vein.
- Fluid in the recesses between the loops.
- Fluid in the peritoneal recesses of the mesentery.
- Free fluid in the peritoneal cavity.

- Due to significant haemorrhagic component, at times, fluid may present some areas with higher attenuation values.
- In small-bowel volvulus, a topographic variation in the position of the bowel loops in the peritoneal cavity takes place, with abnormal spatial configuration and radial shape converging towards the obstruction site. In the same way, the mesenteric vessels show atypical, abnormal course until the inversion of the normal disposition between superior mesenteric artery and vein. The mesenteric vessels are stretched and converge to the obstruction site. Rotation of the bowel and its mesentery depicts the so-called "whirl sign".
- For description of CT findings of the "closed-loop obstruction", we refer the readers to the lecture of E.J. Balthazar (see "Selected Readings").

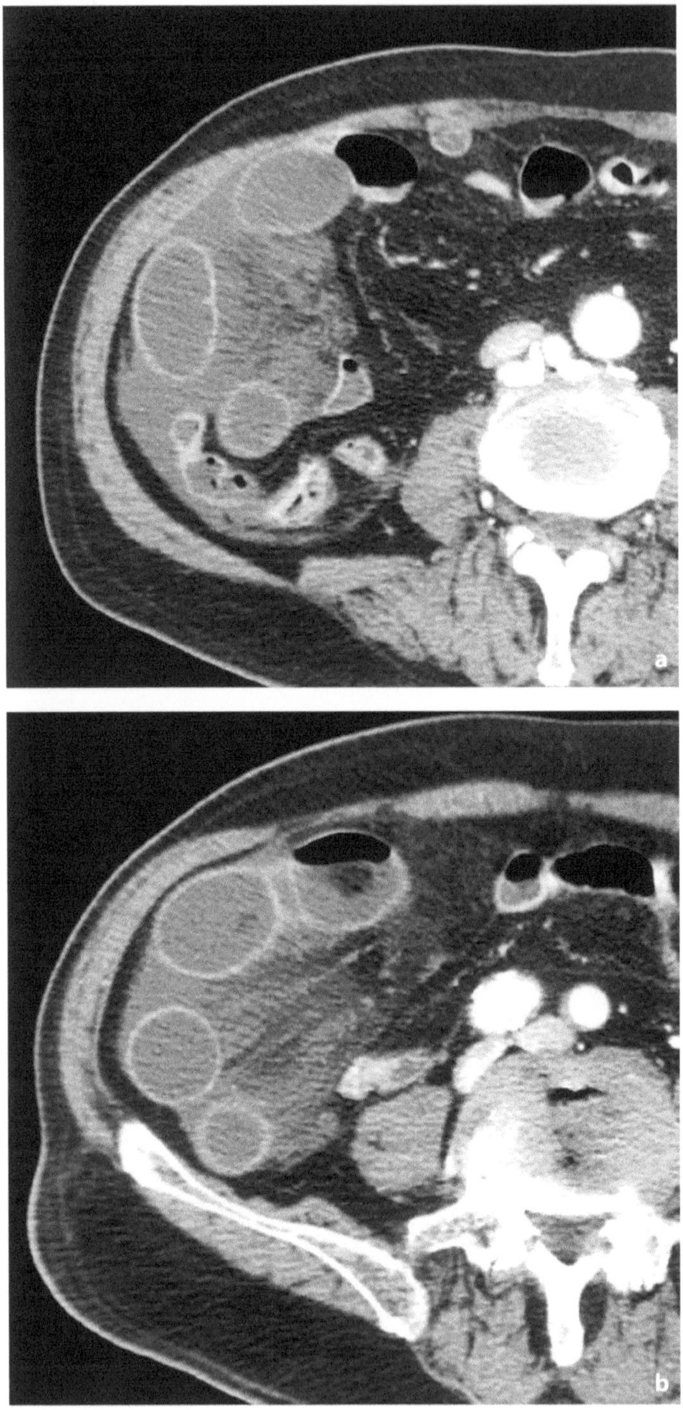

(continue →)

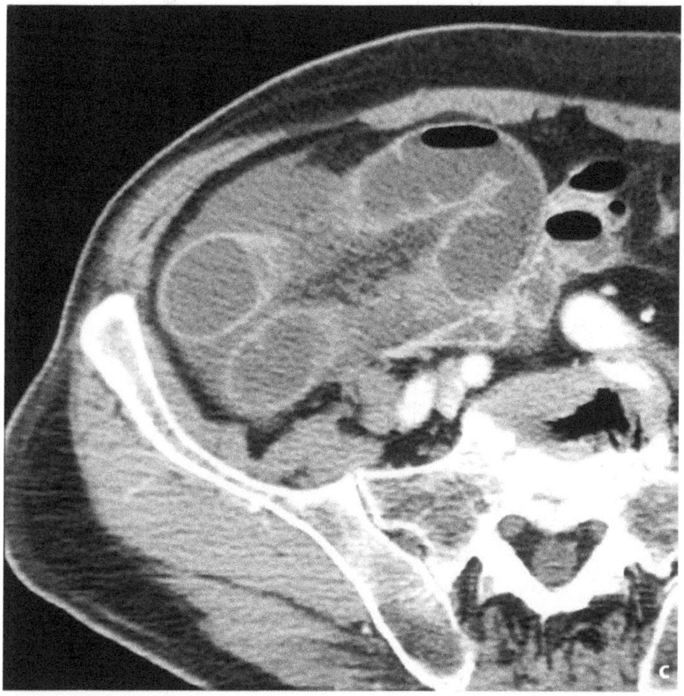

Fig. 3.16 a-c. Complicated small-bowel obstruction due to strangulation. At the opening of the peritoneal cavity, surgery revealed haemoperitoneum and haemorrhage of the mesentery due to ileal volvulus secondary to adhesional band. Resection of 80 cm of ileum. **a-c** Contrast-enhanced multidetector computed tomography (CT). Dilated ileal loops mainly with liquid content. Thin walls with normal and homogeneous contrast enhancement. Opaque inhomogeneous adipose tissue of the adjacent mesentery with transparency loss of the perivascular adipose sheet. Immediate comparison with normal transparency of the adjacent mesentery. High attenuation of the adipose mesenteric tissue may appear before CT finding of pathologic bowel-wall thickening

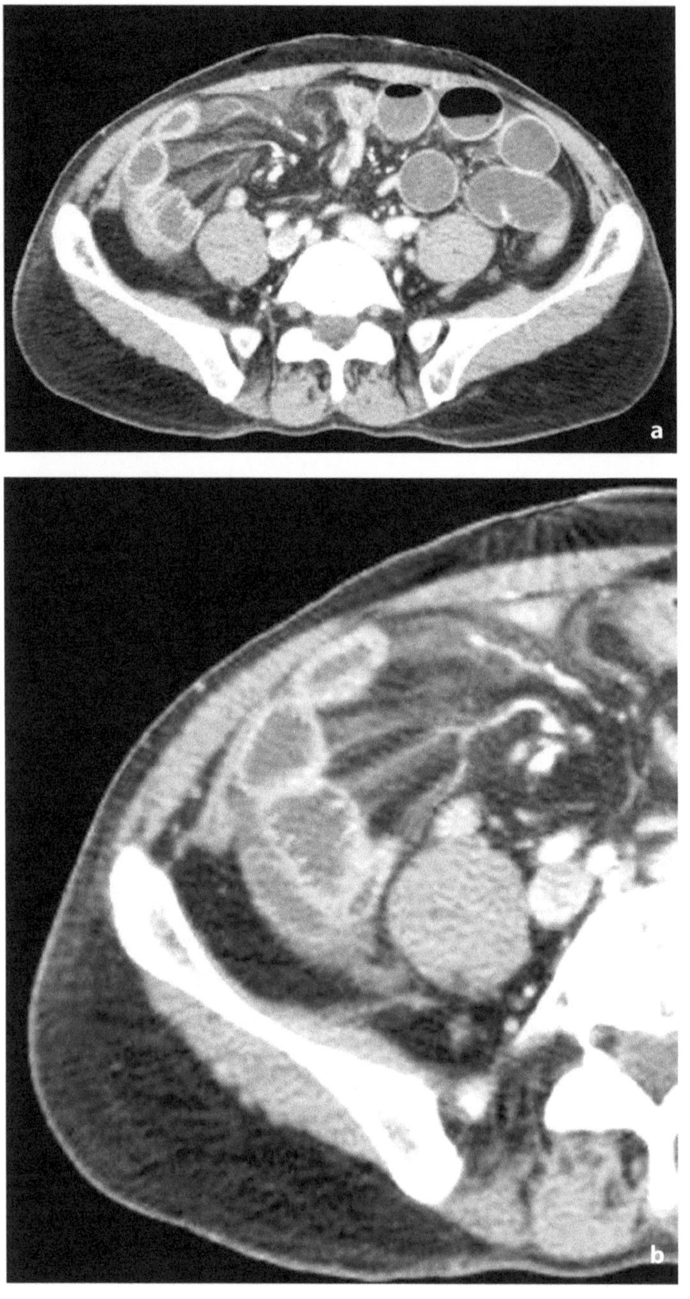

Fig. 3.17 a, b. Complicated small-bowel obstruction due to strangulation. Contrast-enhanced multidetector computed tomography. Initial vascular changes. Dilated small bowel with mainly liquid stasis. In the right iliac fossa, bowel loops with slight wall thickening and increased contrast enhancement. Biological comparison with normal loops located on the left abdominal quadrant is useful. Haziness of the periadventitial adipose sheet surrounding the mesenteric vessels. Small amount of fluid in the peritoneal cavity. Surgery revealed serous-haematic liquid in the peritoneal cavity with small-bowel volvulus by omental band with vascular bowel changes. Resection of the band and volvulus derotation. Tepid water washing and warm, damp patches are used. After a few minutes, restoration of vitality in the injured loops is supported by the reappearance of peristalsis and the progressive recovery of colour

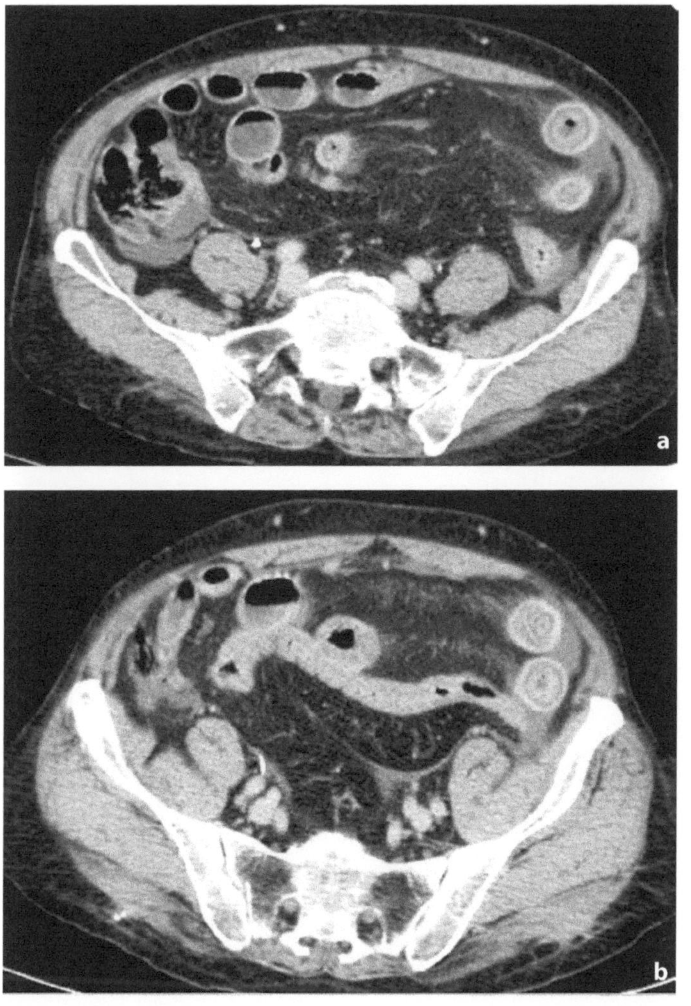

Fig. 3.18 a, b. Complicated small-bowel obstruction due to strangulation. Contrast-enhanced multidetector computed tomography. Thickened bowel and mesentery. Vascular changes of loops in the left iliac fossa and in the middle line characterised by full-thickness bowel wall and prevalence of stratified, target pattern. Haziness of adjacent mesentery. Fluid in the peritoneum. Surgery revealed volvulus with ischaemic necrosis caused by adhesional band. Intestinal resection

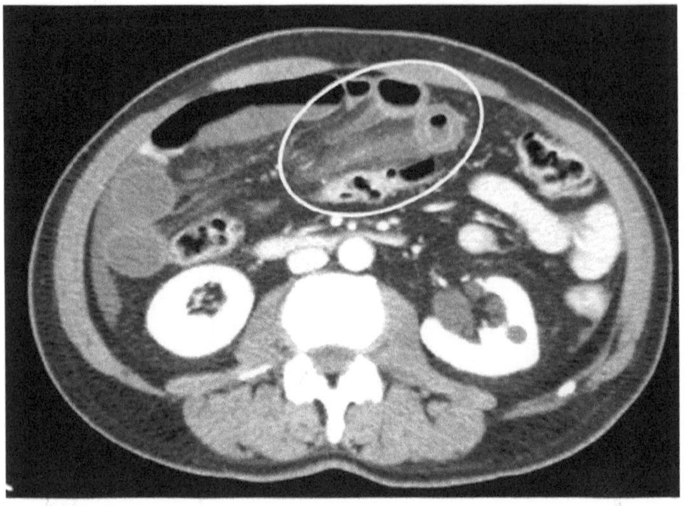

Fig. 3.19. Complicated small-bowel obstruction due to strangulation. Contrast-enhanced multidetector computed tomography. Thickened bowel and focal, circumscribed mesentery (*ellipse*). Stratified bowel-wall thickness with substantially preserved contrast enhancement. Haziness of the perivascular adipose sheet. Peritoneal fluid. Left renal cyst. Segmental volvulus at the transition between jejunum and ileum caused by a band stretched between the omentum and cecum

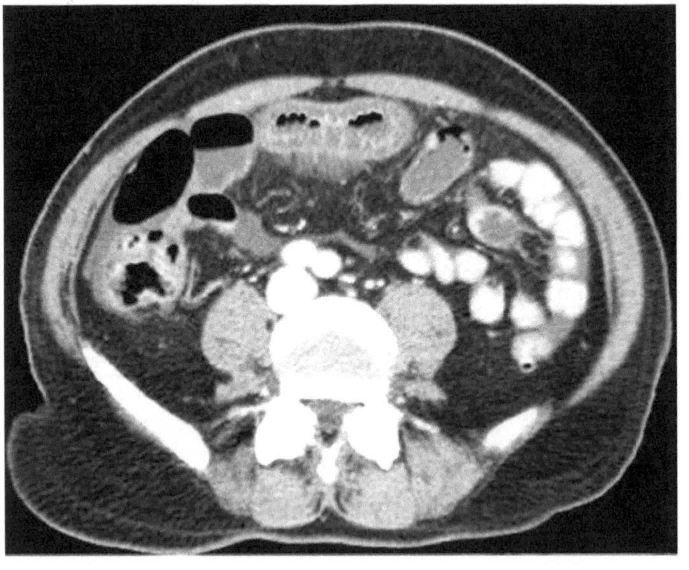

Fig. 3.20. Complicated small-bowel obstruction due to strangulated volvulus secondary to adhesional band. Contrast-enhanced multidetector computed tomography. In the midline, vascular changes of bowel wall are characterised by stratified wall thickness and discrete contrast enhancement, particularly in the inner layer with adjacent dense mesentery. Small amount of fluid in the peritoneal cavity. Band resection and volvulus derotation resolved the obstruction and strangulation. No intestinal resection

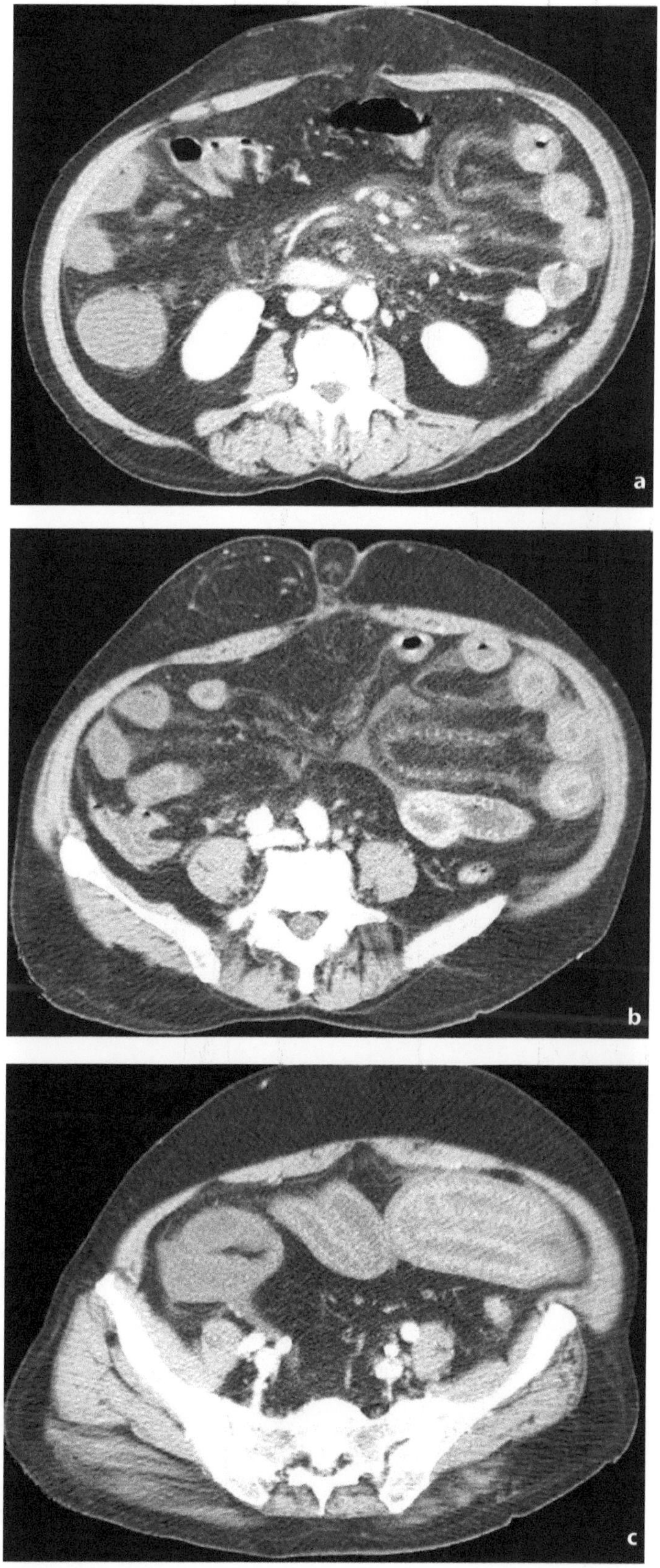

Fig. 3.21 a-c. Complicated small-bowel obstruction due to strangulation. Contrast-enhanced multidetector computed tomography. Thickened bowel and mesentery. **a, b** There are vascular changes of jejunal loops with marked full thickness of the bowel walls. Mild contrast enhancement tending to stratification. Haziness of the perivascular adipose sheet surrounding the mesenteric vessels is clearly evident. The mesenteric root is also cloudy and misty. At the level of the mesenteric recesses, free fluid tends to pool, creating a bizarre shape. Median incisional hernia. **c** More caudally, vascular changes of the loops in longitudinal view

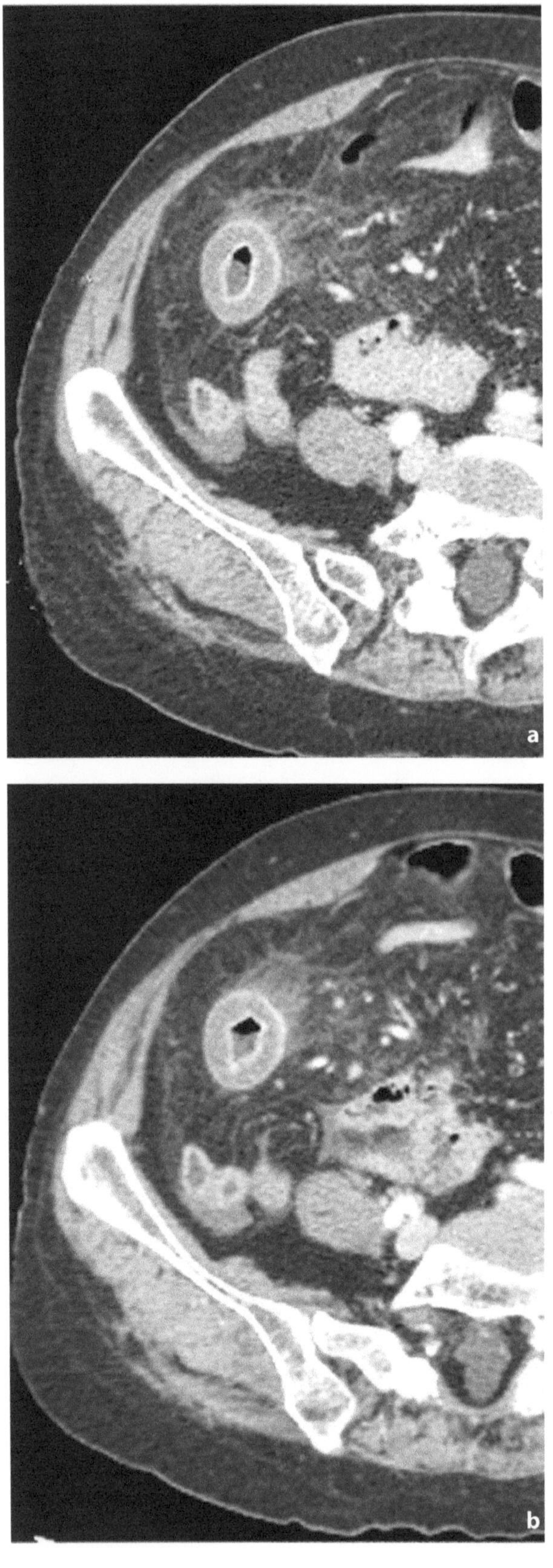

Fig. 3.22 a-d. Complicated small-bowel obstruction due to strangulated volvulus. Contrast-enhanced multidetector computed tomography. Particulars of the right iliac fossa. Full-thickness loop with vascular changes. Stratified pattern with target shape: the inner and outer rings are thin, with elevated contrast enhancement. The middle ring is uniformly and markedly thick and relatively hypodense. Moderate lumen distension with liquid–gaseous content. The adjacent mesentery is thick, blurred and opaque: engorgement and congestion of the adjacent mesenteric circle. Moderate amount of peritoneal fluid. Surgery revealed haemoperitoneum and ileal volvulus due to adhesional band. Deeply ischaemic bowel loop, whose colour is mainly black anthracite. Surgical resection of about 15 cm of small intestine (*cont.* →)

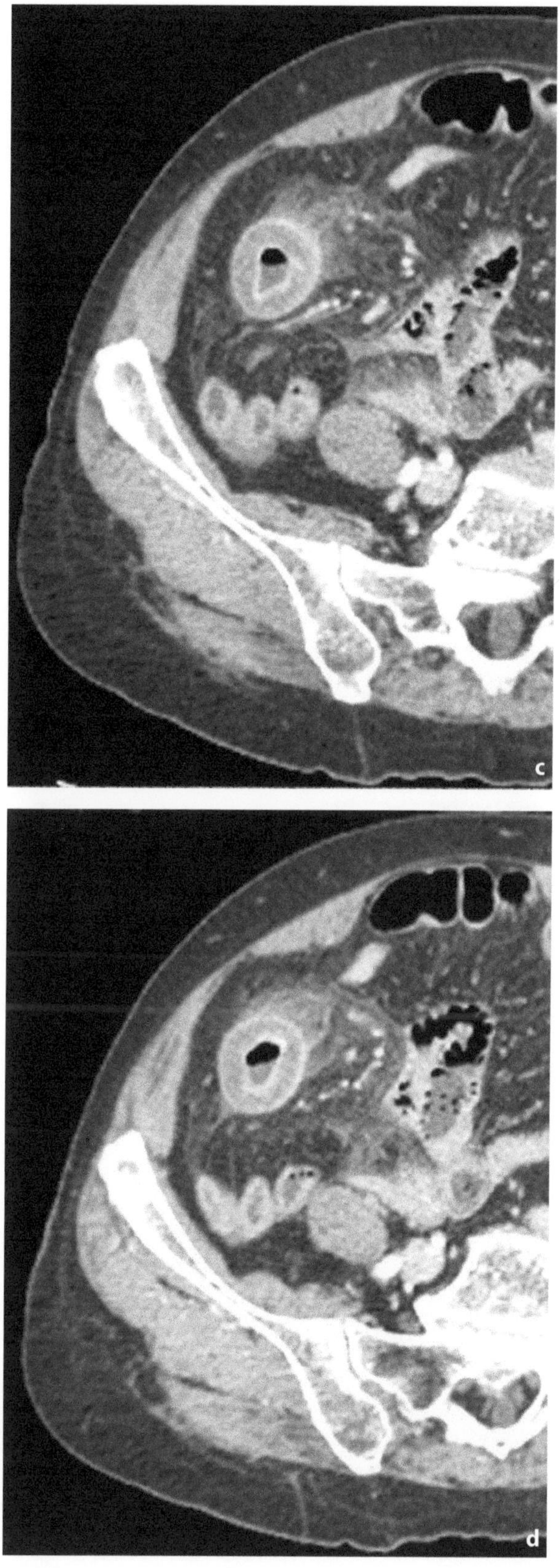
c
d

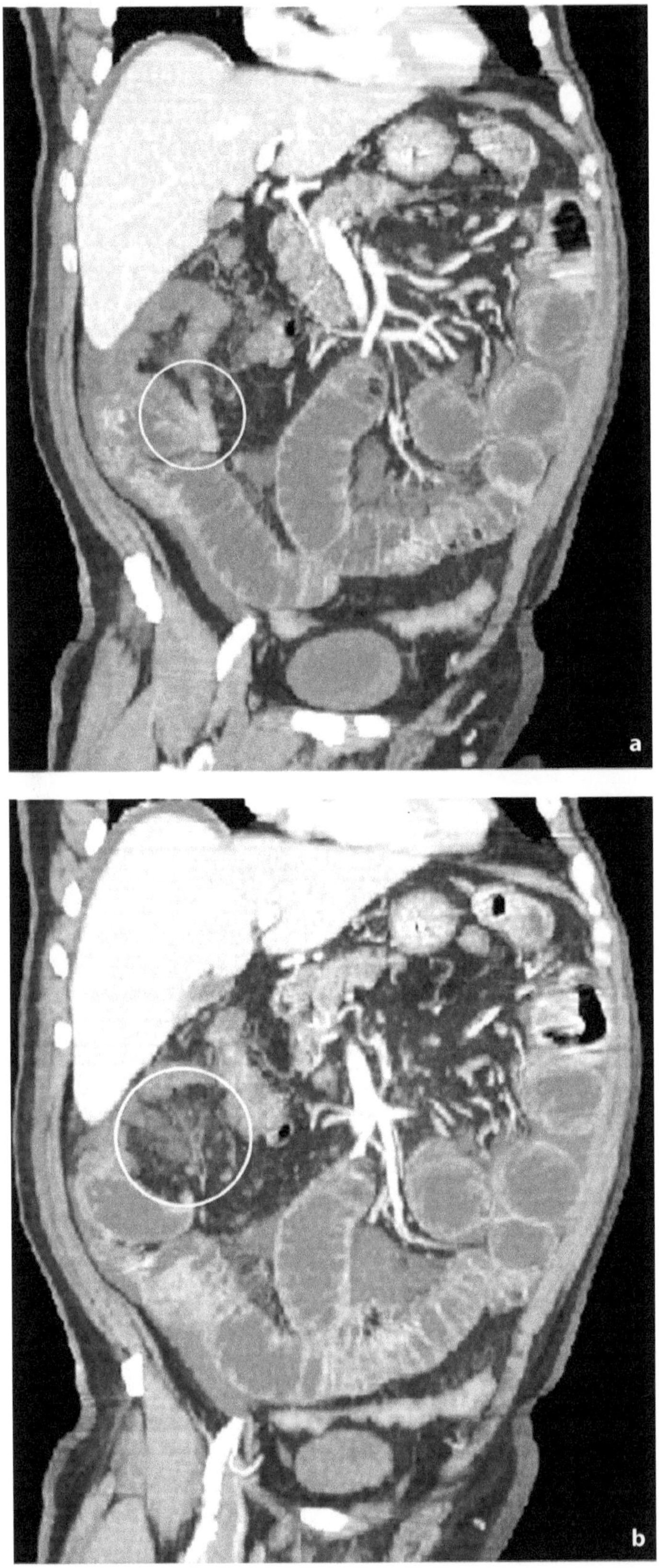

(cont. →)

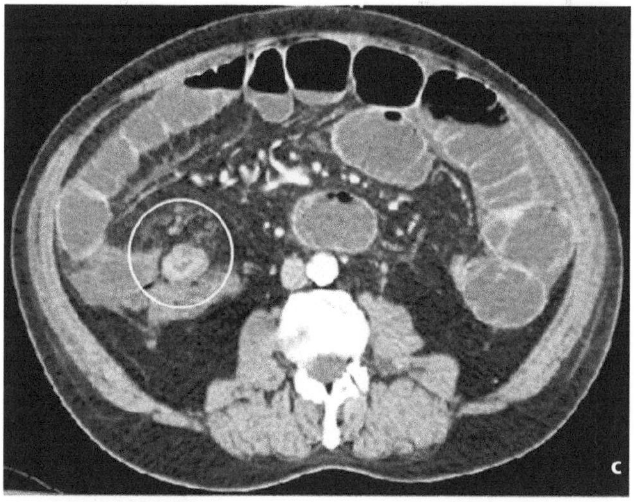

Fig. 3.23 a-c. Complicated small-bowel obstruction due to strangling. A complex mechanism is the cause of obstruction. Surgery revealed a carcinoma in the ascending colon, with deep ulceration. The ulcerative process caused circular erosion of the adjacent omental apron, with a subsequent wide fissure. In this peritoneal neocavity, a small-bowel loop is herniated and strangled. Contrast-enhanced multidetector computed tomography. **a, b** Multiplanar reconstruction combined with maximum intensity projection on oblique coronal planes. Proximal ileal–jejunal obstruction. Below the inferior hepatic margin, a loop herniated into a peritoneal neocavity is visible. The neck of the hernia in (**a**) (*circle*) is narrow and compresses both the afferent and the efferent segment, determining a closed loop at two adjacent point of its arch. The mesentery of the herniated loop is blurred and hazy in (**b**) (*circle*). Peritoneal fluid. **c** Axial scan at the level of the herniated loop. Vascular changes of the loop with parietal stratified thickness (*circle*). Contrast enhancement substantially preserved. As a biological parameter for assessment, comparison with the remaining obstructed loops without vascular changes is useful. Partial omentectomy and right hemicolectomy

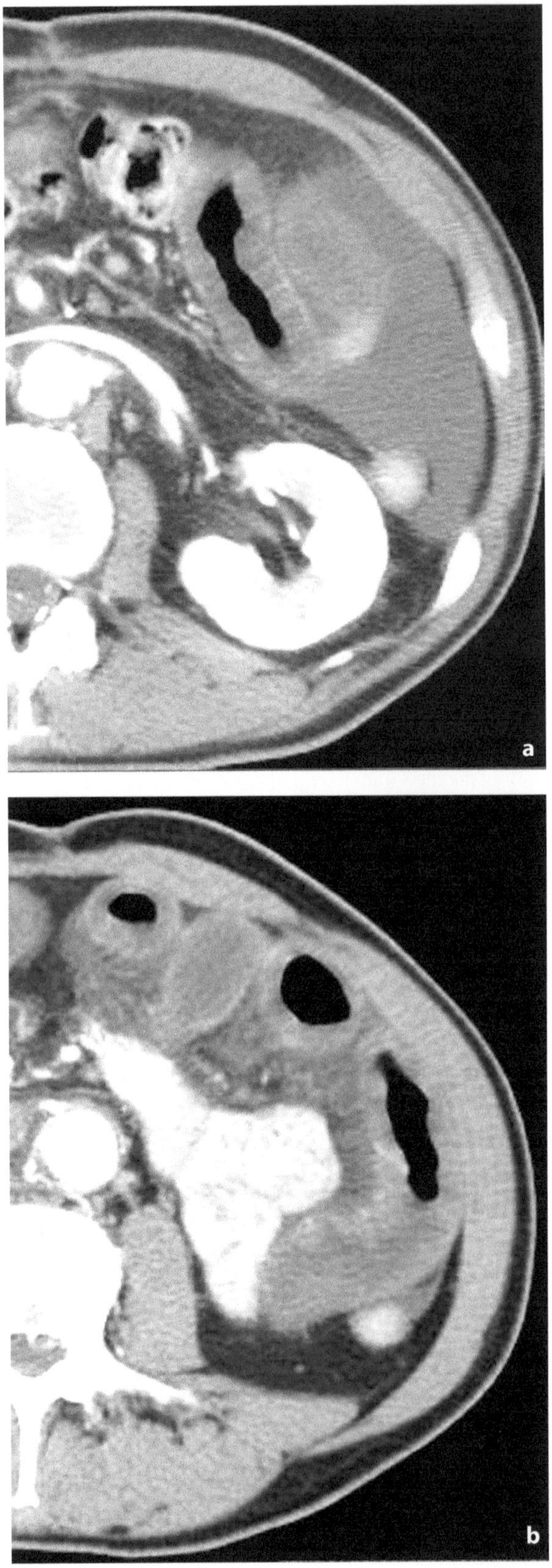

(cont. →)

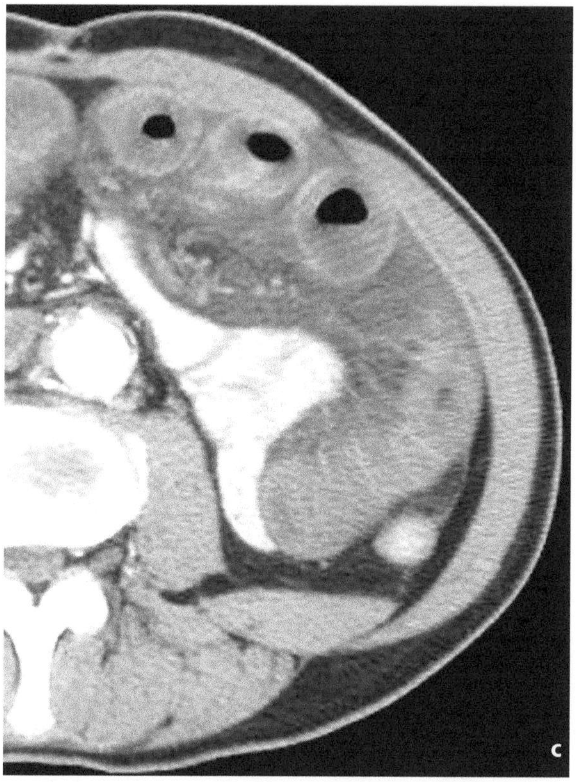

Fig. 3.24 a-c. Complicated small-bowel obstruction due to strangulation. Contrast-enhanced multidetector computed tomography. **a** Jejunal loop with vascular changes showing marked parietal thickness and mild to scarce contrast enhancement (CE). Limited lumen distension. Abundant amount of peritoneal fluid. **b, c** Detail of left flank. Thickened loops with scarce or absent CE. Mild lumen distension. Thickened mesentery diffusely and deeply opaque. Peritoneal fluid. Loops distal to the obstruction site, collapsed and crowded, with preserved CE. Surgery revealed ileal–jejunal volvulus due to adhesional band with serrated strangulation. Wide intestinal resection

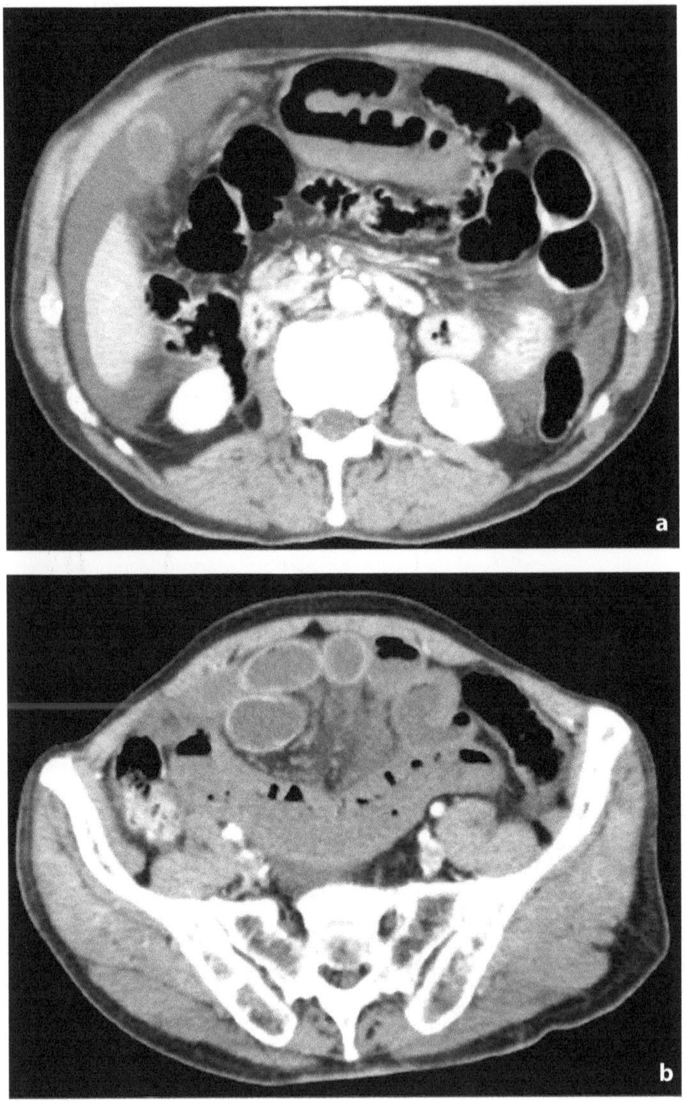

Fig. 3.25 a,b. Complicated small-bowel obstruction due to strangulation. Contrast-enhanced multidetector computed tomography. **a** At the middle line, rigid, thickened jejunal loop without parietal stratification and without contrast enhancement (CE). Liquid–gaseous stasis. Abundant amount of peritoneal fluid. **b** Posteriorly, a thickened loop without stratification or CE is visible. The rigid loop has lost its morphology and tone. Mainly liquid stasis. As a biological parameter for assessment, comparison with the remaining obstructed loops without vascular changes is useful. Misty and opaque mesentery. Peritoneal fluid. Surgery revealed strangulation by volvulus with necrosis. Intestinal resection

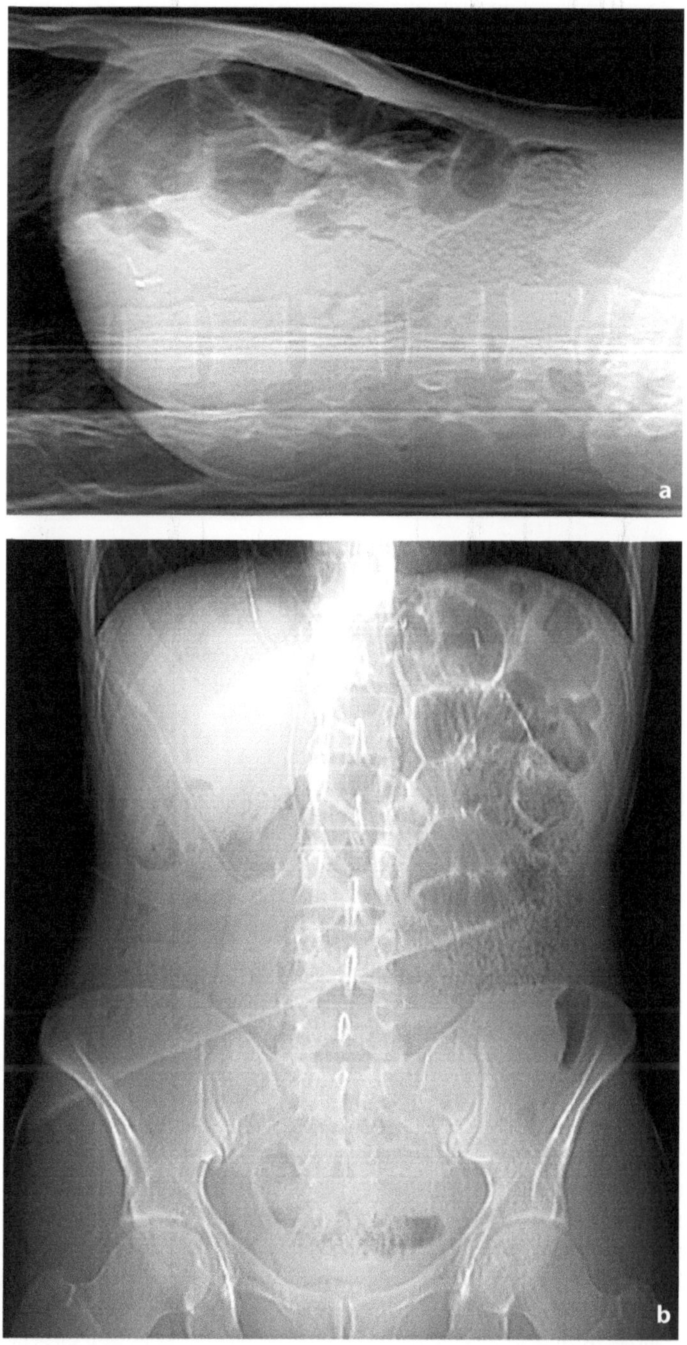

Fig. 3.26 a-h. Complicated small-bowel obstruction due to strangulation. Contrast-enhanced multidetector computed tomography. **a, b** Frontal and lateral scout views. Positioning of the nasogastric tube reduced the liquid component of stasis. The luminal content is condensed, mimicking the presence of faeces in the small bowel. Gas distends the first jejunal loops, showing numerous and crowded valvulae conniventes. The remaining abdominal quadrants are mainly opaque and therefore mask bowel-wall features. (*cont.* →)

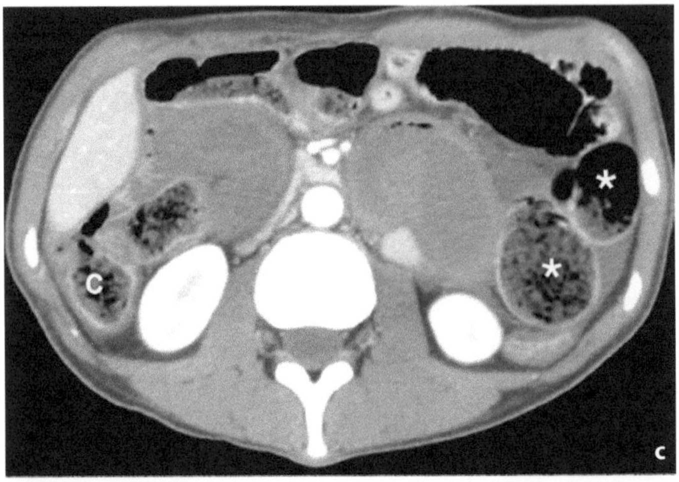

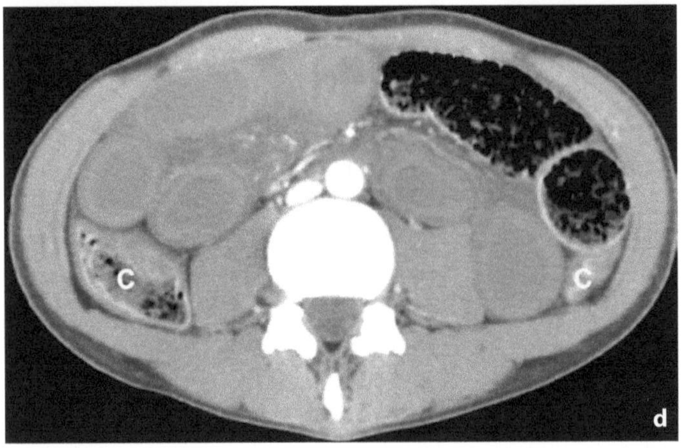

c Scan passing through the inferior margin of the liver. *Asterisks* indicate distended loops with thin walls and preserved contrast enhancement (CE), without vascular changes; gaseous and faecaloid stasis. At both sides of the median line, ischaemic dilated loops with mainly liquid content, thickened walls, without CE, are visible. Peritoneal fluid. *C* identifies the right colon with faecal content and normal CE. **d** Scan passing through the medium abdomen. On the left, dilated small-bowel loops with faecal-like content, without vascular changes. The remaining fluid-filled loops of the small intestine are deeply ischaemic: full-thickness walls without CE. The adipose tissue of the mesentery is diffusely opaque. Peritoneal fluid. *C*, colon. **e** *White circle* indicates the transition zone as abrupt diameter change between the dilated and the collapsed loops. Distal to the obstruction site, collapsed terminal ileum with normal CE is visible. *Black circle* identifies the ileocecal junction. **f** Scan passing through the iliac wings. Arterial spasm, with reduction in the number and diameter of vessels, is visible. Opaque mesentery. The loops are deeply ischaemic. Peritoneal fluid. *C*, colon. **g**, **h** Multiplanar reconstruction on oblique coronal planes. The following features are visible: spasm of the superior mesenteric artery branches (**g**); opaque mesentery, strangulated and volvulus loops with spiral disposition (**h**); non-ischaemic distended proximal jejunum; peritoneal fluid. Surgery revealed massive ileal volvulus due to adhesional band with massive necrosis. Subtotal enterectomy (*cont.* →)

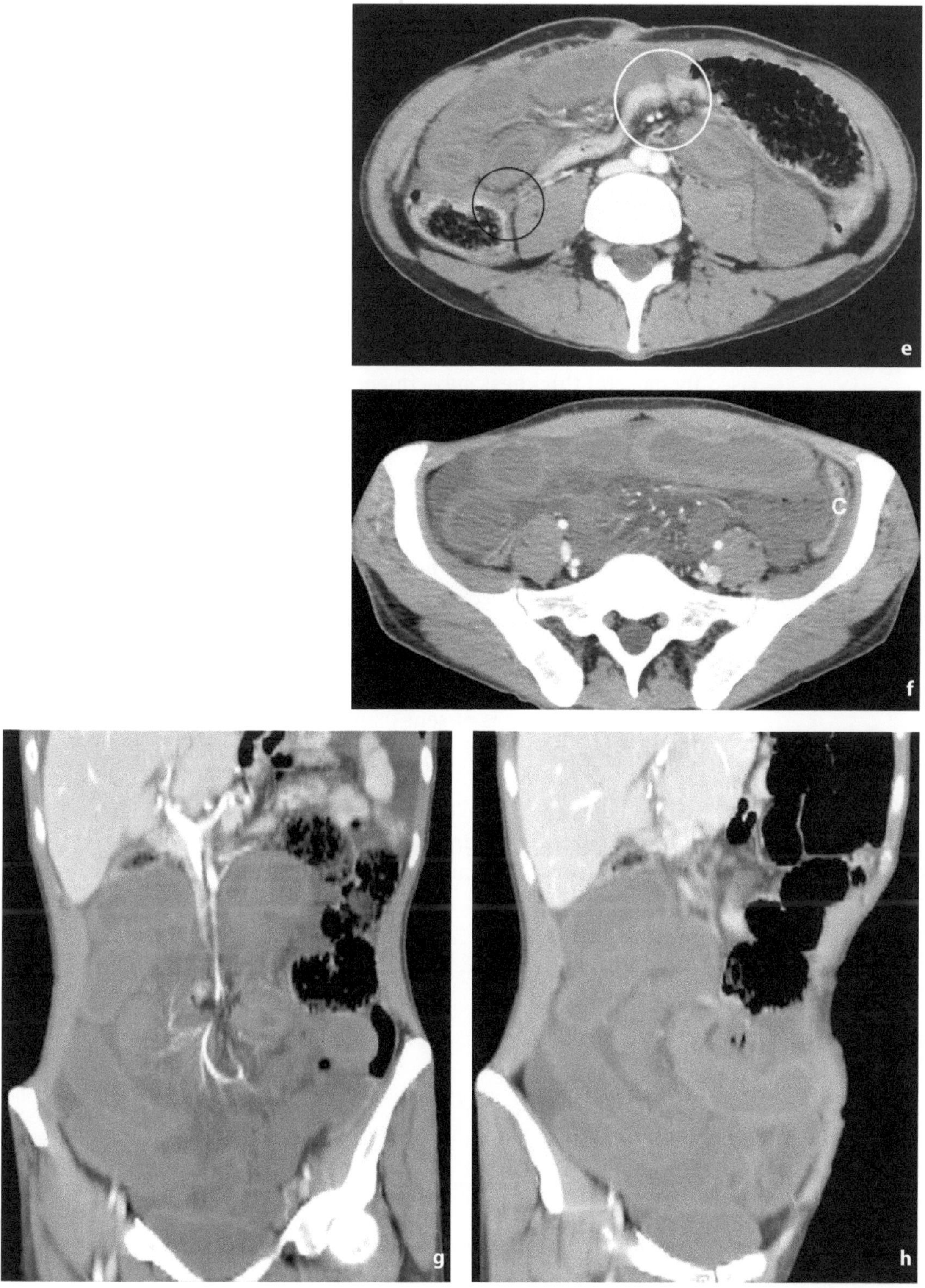
e
C
f
g
h

Complicated SBO due to Fight

Thickened Bowel Images (Figs. 3.27 and 3.28)

Loop vascular changes due to fight may complicate simple or decompensated SBO. Changes due to fight determine iconographic abnormalities of wall density and thickness.

Mesenteric involvement is absent or minimal. These confined changes add to CT features of simple and decompensated SBO:

- Usually, loop due to fight is close to the obstruction site and is characterised by parietal thickness subsequent to venous stasis. Loop CE due to fight is higher in comparison with that of the remaining loops. At the onset of complicated SBO, parietal thickness is preserved or borderline. Actually, loop due to fight appears dense first and then thickens. As a consequence, a pattern of thickened and hyperdense loop with homogeneous shape and without stratification is evident. This thickening and CE change are primarily related to the mesenteric border of the loops. Evaluation of initial thickness is subjective: comparison with the adjacent loops is a useful biological parameter. Vascular changes in a loop due to fight have an intrinsic evolution, which may determine alteration of early parietal pattern.
- Mesenteric involvement is absent or minimal. Abnormality of the confluent fascia loop mesentery may be evident. These late findings are evidence of slowing and stasis in the mesenteric vasculature, restricted to affected bowel segment. Vessel dilatation and mesenteric haziness are visible and limited to the confluent fascia loop mesentery.
- Free fluid in the peritoneal cavity is frequently present.

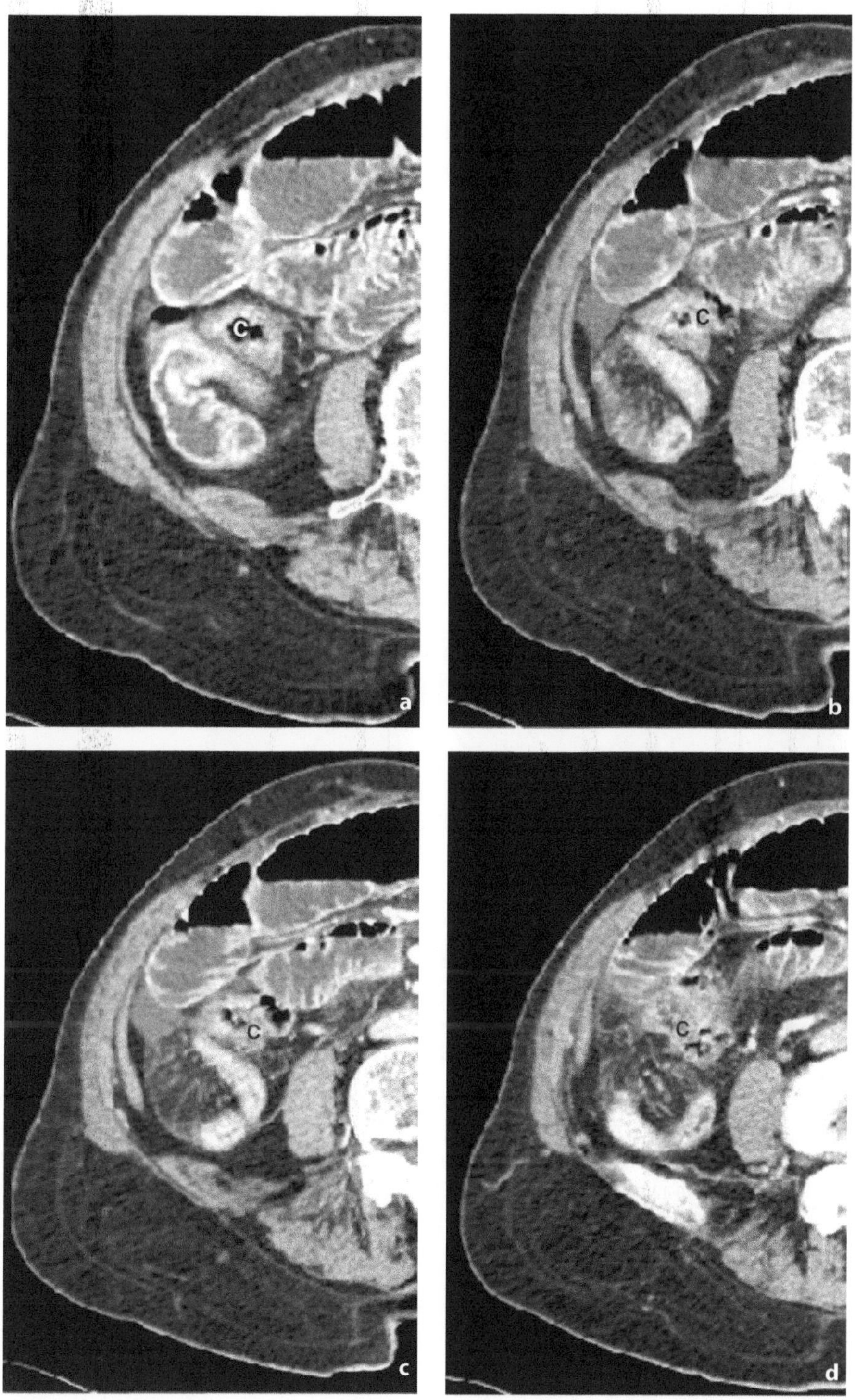

Fig. 3.27 a-d. Complicated small-bowel obstruction due to fight. Surgery revealed mobile cecum, and ischaemic last ileal loop incarcerated into internal hernia of retrocecal recess. Contrast-enhanced multidetector computed tomography. Thickened bowel images. **a** A tract of terminal ileum shows mild wall thickness at the mesenteric border. The antimesenteric border shows borderline thickness. Parietal contrast enhancement (CE) is uniformly increased. *C*, cecum. **b-d** Encapsulated and fixed aspect of the terminal ileum, which presents a full-thickness wall, with increased and homogeneous CE without stratification. The herniated mesentery is transparent. Normal vascularity. Small amount of peritoneal fluid. *C*, cecum. Surgical reduction of the incarcerated loop allowed restoration of its viability

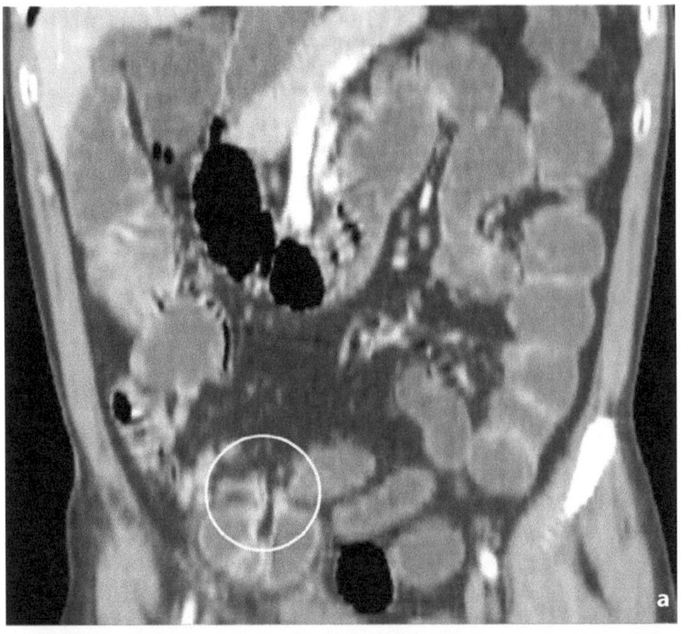

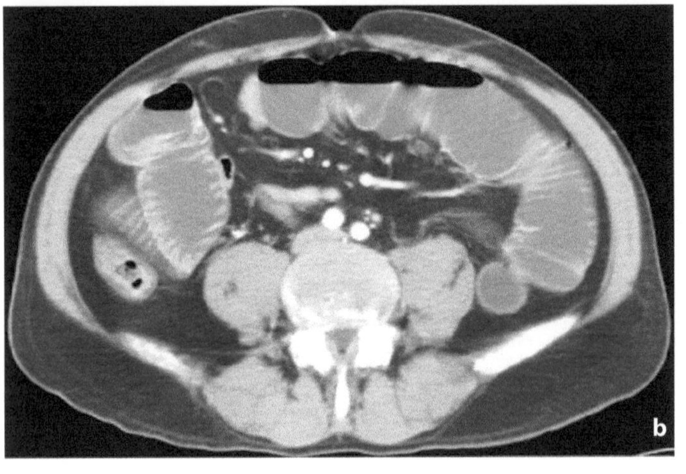

Fig. 3.28 a-d. Complicated small-bowel obstruction due to fight. Right paravesical hernia with incarcerated loop. Contrast-enhanced multidetector computed tomography after hydric distension of the large bowel. **a** Oblique coronal multiplanar reconstruction . Distal ileal–jejunal distension. At the right hemipelvis, a closed loop herniated into an anomalous recess is evident. *Circle* identifies hernia orifice. **b** Scan through lower abdomen. Distended small bowel with preserved parietal–valvular features. Liquid–gaseous stasis. Normotransparent mesentery. Normal vascularity. (*cont.* →)

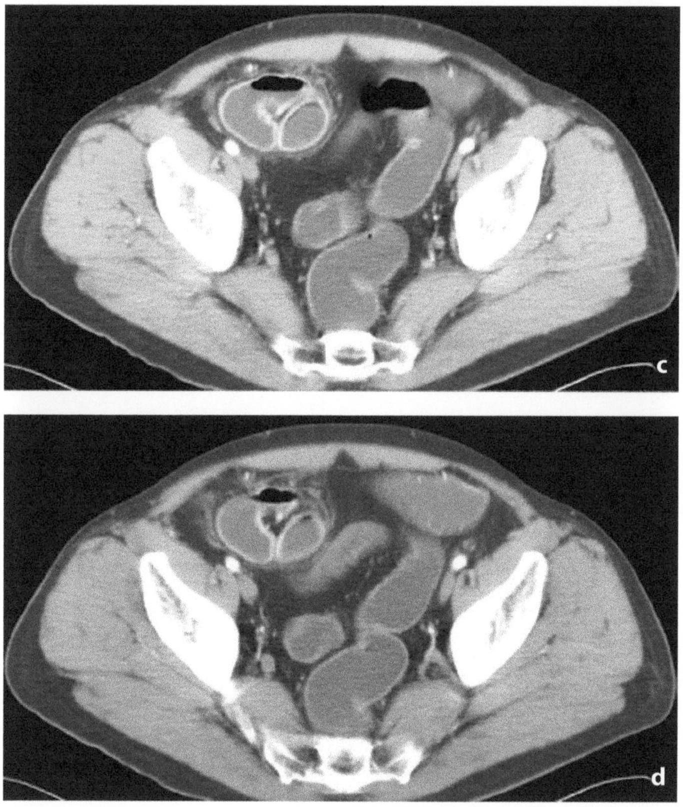

c, d Scans passing through the pelvis. There is a loop with a collected, encapsulated and fixed aspect in the peritoneal cavity is seen. The herniated loop is in vascular changes due to fight: borderline parietal thickness with increased contrast enhancement. Immediately useful is biological comparison with the other loops of the small and large bowel. The mesentery of the herniated loop is transparent, and the perivascular adipose sheet is preserved. After tepid-water washings and the application of warm, damp patches, the injured loop regained vitality

4 Sonographic Correlations

R. Di Mizio, V. Di Mizio, G. Annunziata, R. Cianci, A. Filippone

When small-bowel obstruction (SBO) is suspected, we usually perform an ultrasound (US) of the small bowel in order to correlate the results with those of the abdominal plain film. US is able to not only confirm and support the initial diagnosis, it also offers additional findings and enhances the overall diagnostic confidence.

Main US features arise from the assessment of fluid-filled bowel loops and the identification of peritoneal fluid. This evidence is helpful when integrating conventional plain films, which mainly depict the features of air-filled intestinal loops, being unable to analyse the fluid-filled bowel. On the other hand, fluid acts as an acoustic window for US, which is able to assess the diameter and the wall of the distended loops. US is highly sensitive in detection of peritoneal fluid but nonspecific in defining its nature. The real-time assessment also allows evaluation of bowel motility.

The limitation of US is mainly due to its inability to provide adequate information on the involvement of the mesentery (Figs. 4.1–4.10).

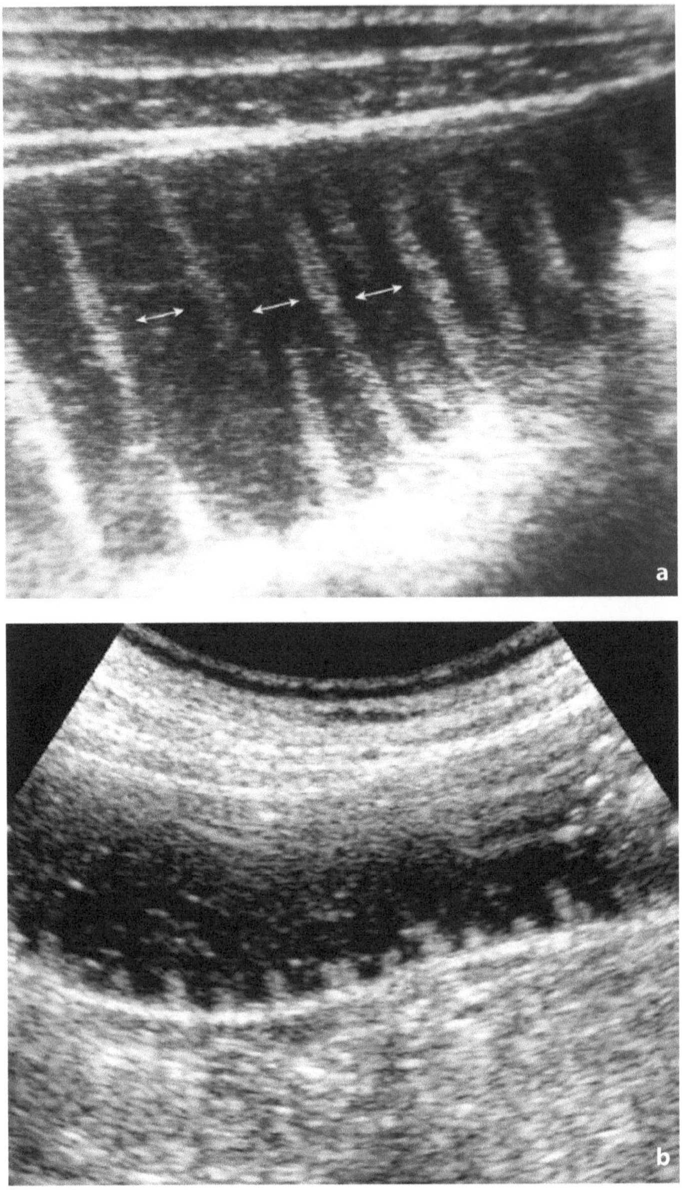

Fig. 4.1 a, b. Simple small-bowel obstruction. Sonography in two patients performed with linear small parts probe (**a**) and abdominal convex probe (**b**). Dilated jejunal loops with liquid content. Normal and thin walls. Numerous and preserved valvulae conniventes (*arrows*). Absence of peritoneal fluid (Fig. 4.1a from Grassi R et al. (2004) The relevance of free fluid between intestinal loops detected by sonography in the clinical assessment of small-bowel obstruction in adults. Eur J Radiol 50:5–14, reproduced with permission)

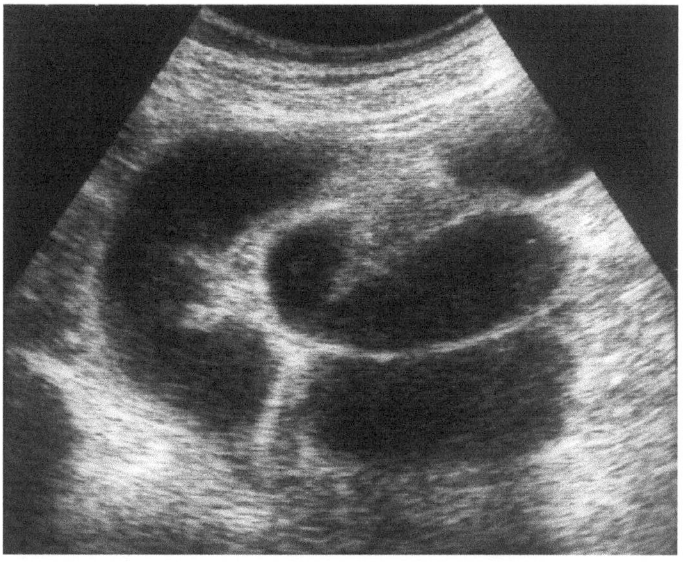

Fig. 4.2. Simple small-bowel obstruction. Sonography. Dilated ileal loops with liquid content. Thin walls. Flattened valvulae conniventes by increased intraluminal tension. Absence of peritoneal fluid

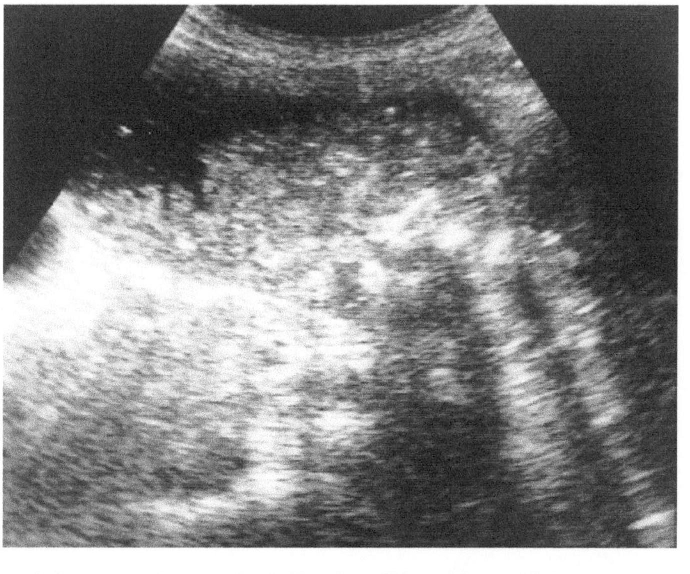

Fig. 4.3. Simple small-bowel obstruction. Sonography. A dilated small-bowel loop with heterogeneous content, mimicking faecal material

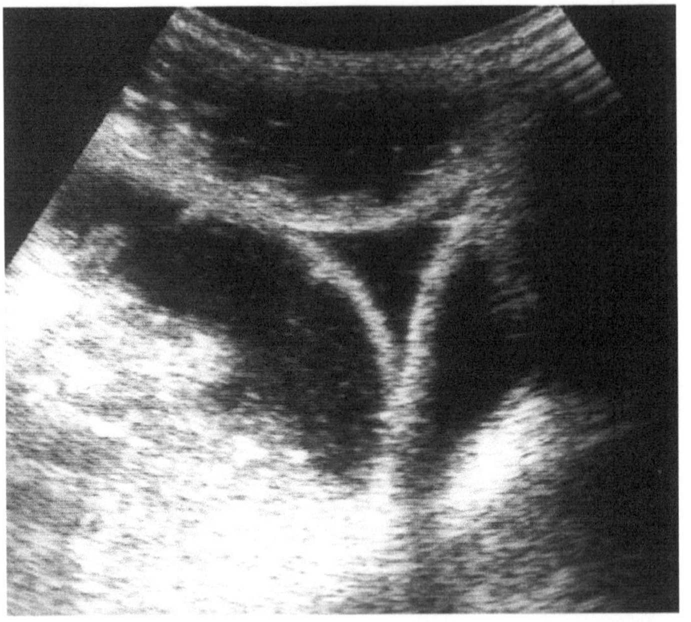

Fig. 4.4. Decompensated small-bowel obstruction. Sonography. Dilated ileal loops with liquid content. Thin walls. Free fluid in recesses between loops assumes typical triangular shape (tanga sign) (From Grassi R et al. (2004) The relevance of free fluid between intestinal loops detected by sonography in the clinical assessment of small bowel obstruction in adults. Eur J Radiol 50:5–14, reproduced with permission)

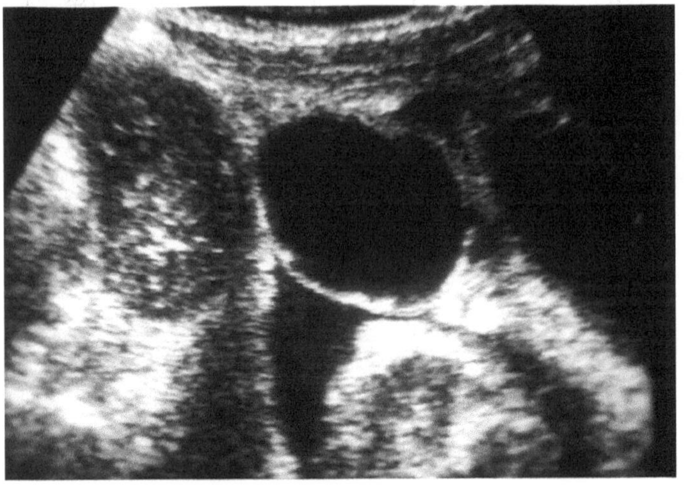

Fig. 4.5. Decompensated small-bowel obstruction. Sonography. Dilated ileal loops with different content, both echogenic and anechogenic. Thin walls. Fluid forms typical triangular shape (tanga sign)

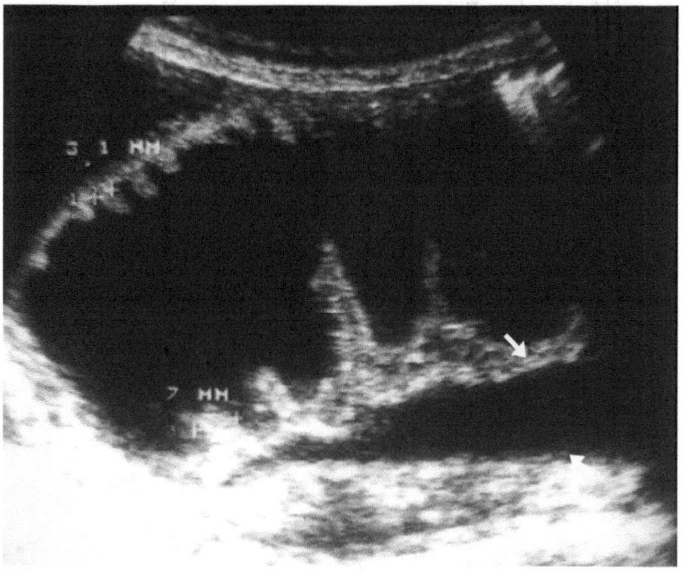

Fig. 4.6. Complicated small-bowel obstruction. Sonography. Dilated jejunal loop with liquid content. Echogenic, heterogeneous fold and bowel-wall thickening, particularly visible on the mesenteric border. Mesenteric border folds achieve 7-mm versus 3.1-mm thickness of antimesenteric border folds. Peritoneal fluid (*arrows*). Mesenteric findings are poor (From Di Mizio R et al. (1995) Ileo meccanico "scompensato" dell'intestino tenue nell'adulto. Radiol Med 89:787–791, reproduced with permission)

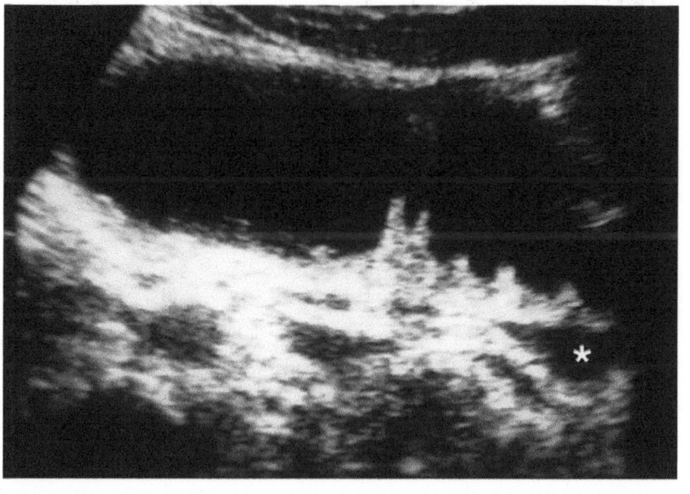

Fig. 4.7. Complicated small-bowel obstruction. Sonography. Dilated ileal loops with liquid content. Asymmetric, echogenic, essentially homogeneous fold and bowel-wall thickening, restricted to the mesenteric border. Free fluid in the peritoneal cavity (*asterisk*)

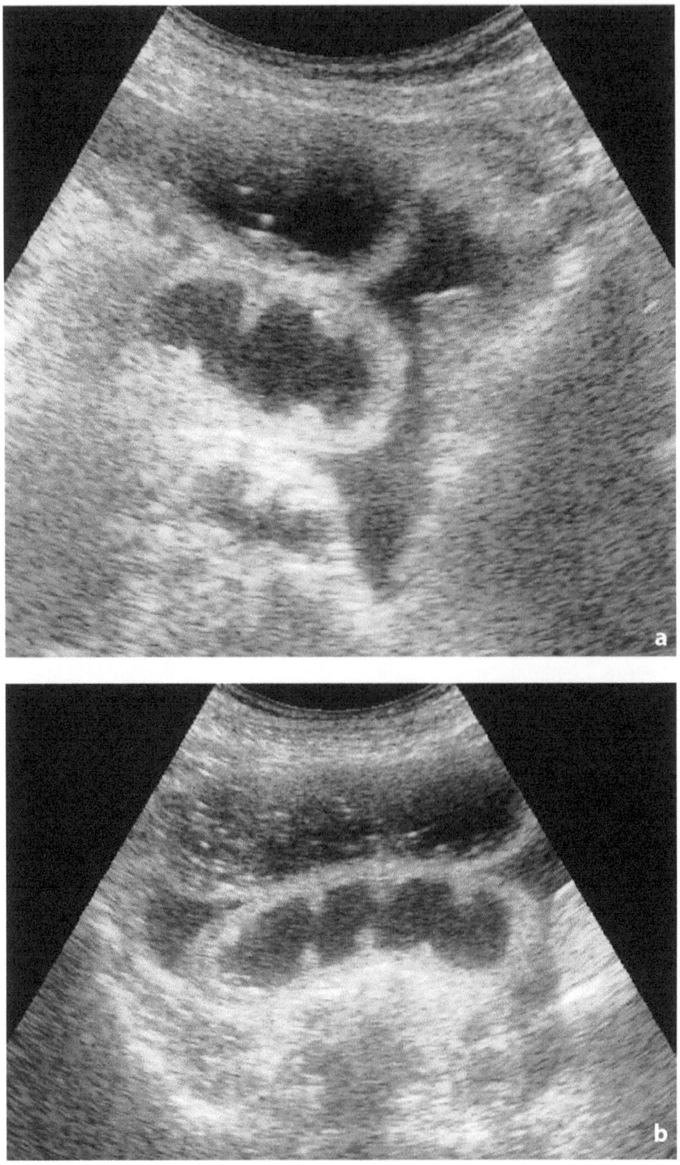

Fig. 4.8 a, b. Complicated small-bowel obstruction. Sonography. Posterior loop presents echogenic, homogeneous and marked fold and bowel-wall thickening at the entire circumference without stratification. Large amount of free fluid in the peritoneal cavity. Mesenteric findings are poor

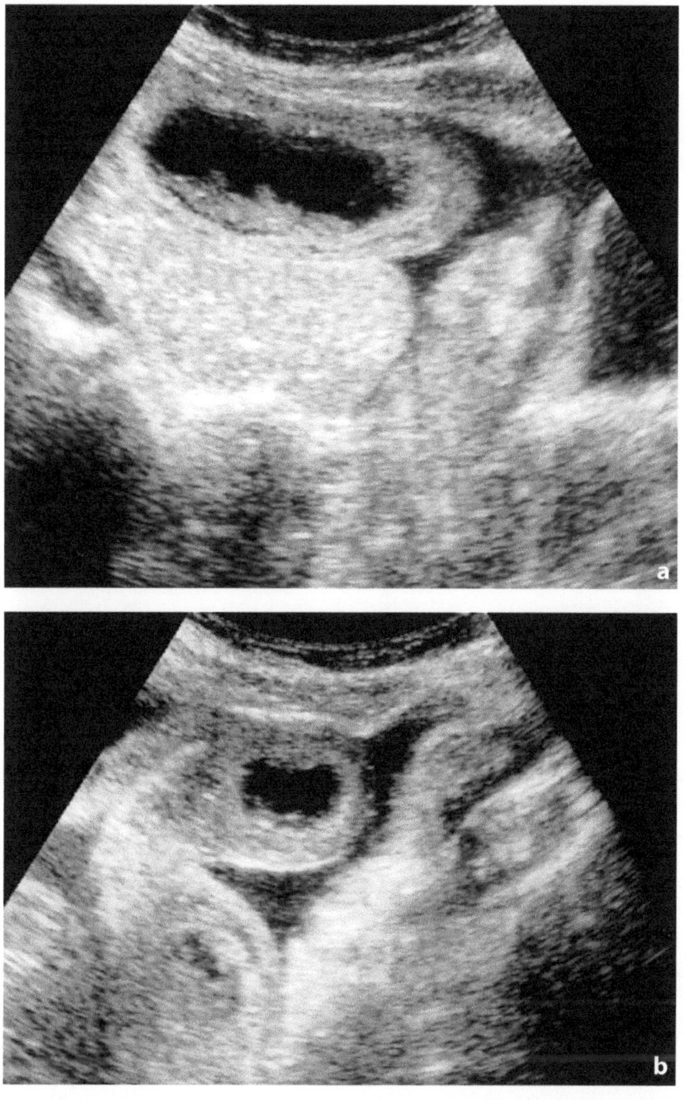

Fig. 4.9 a, b. Complicated small-bowel obstruction. Sonography. Anterior loop is moderately dilated, with mainly liquid content. Echogenic and marked bowel-wall thickening at the entire circumference, at times mildly heterogeneous, without stratification. Fluid forms typical triangular shape (tanga sign). Mesenteric findings are poor

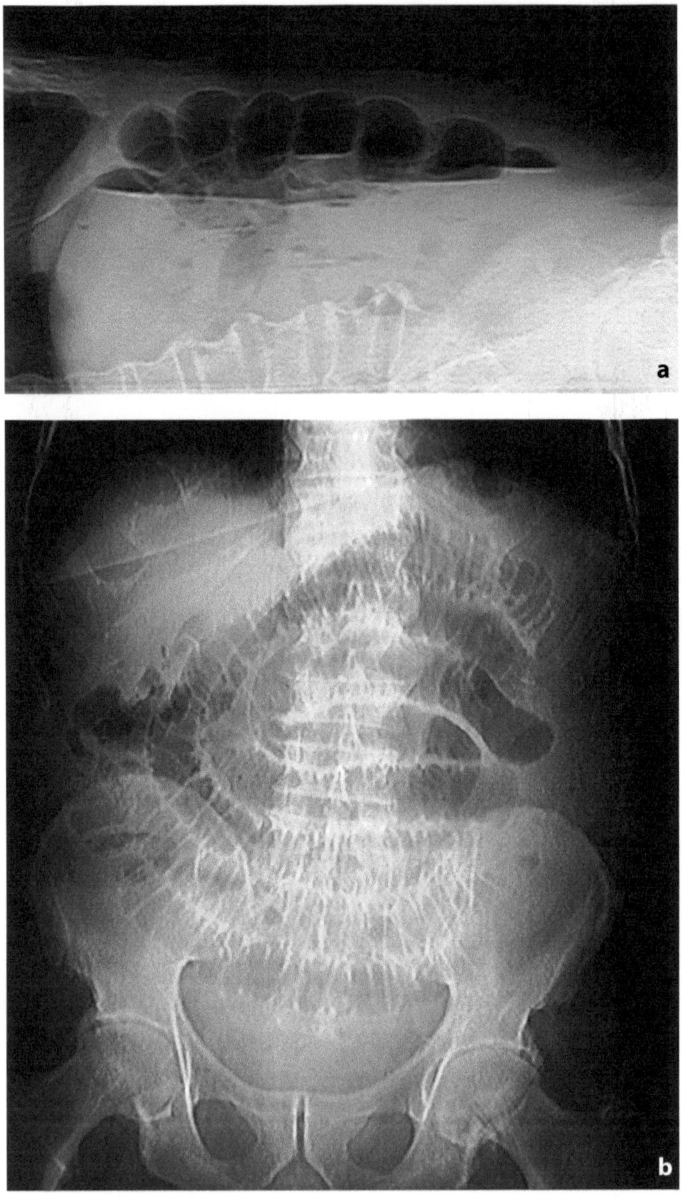

Fig. 4.10 a-c. Complicated small-bowel obstruction (SBO). Radiographic and sonographic integration. **a, b** Frontal and lateral abdominal views in digital films. Marked ileal–jejunal distension with mixed enteric stasis. Colic frame barely detectable. Numerous and forced valvulae conniventes. Loops with mainly gaseous content show thin walls. (*cont.* →)

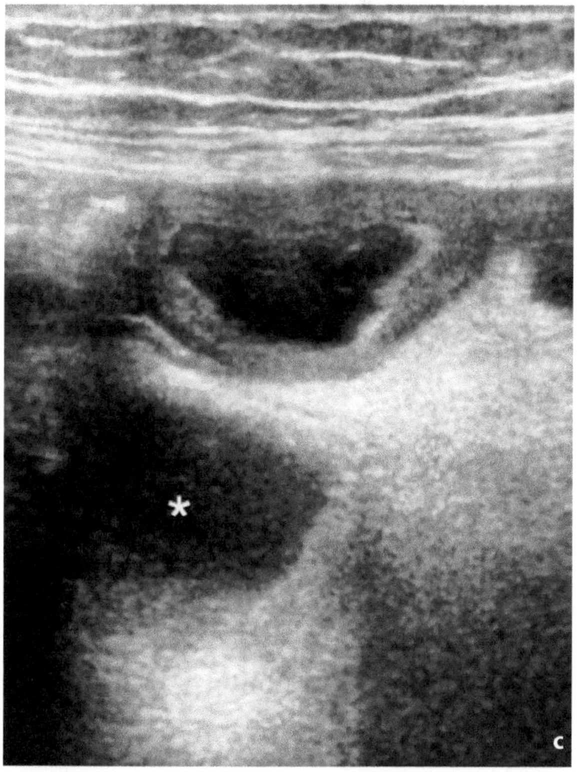

c Sonographic integration reveals both free fluid in the peritoneal cavity (*asterisk*) and concentric wall thickening of fluid-filled bowel loop in the right iliac fossa. Sonography confirms and supports radiographic diagnosis of SBO. Furthermore, it shows findings of vascular changes of strangling loop into internal hernia of retrocecal recess. Mesentery status difficult to evaluate

5 Radiological Correlations

R. Di Mizio, V. Di Mizio, R. Della Marra, D. Di Rocco, R. Sciarra, R. Grassi

The new imaging modalities have changed the role of conventional radiology in the study of the acute abdomen. Nevertheless, the abdominal plain film can still be used:

- in searching for radiopaque foreign bodies;
- in identifying free intraperitoneal air;
- in postsurgical follow-up;
- in the study of acute intestinal behaviours.

Examination Technique

Prior to the abdominal plain film, it is advisable to:

- Avoid cleansing enema: the introduction of water causes image interference, which may be misleading.
- Delay the introduction of nasogastric or rectal catheters, as they tend to reduce gastrointestinal stasis, which is important for morphological and diagnostic orientation.
- Know the type and duration of drug treatment, given its ability to modify intestinal tone and motility.

In intestinal occlusions, intraluminal stasis with various amounts of air component develops. This condition causes a strong contrast difference between the radiolucency of intestinal air and the slight radiopacity of abdominal soft tissue. This difference of contrast values should not be increased. Therefore, abdominal plain films have to be performed with low milliampere and medium to high kilovolt values. This approach will give a soft representation of all abdominal and intestinal components.

Uncooperative Patient

The ill patient with acute abdomen may be cooperative or uncooperative. In case of the uncooperative patient, two overview radiographs of the abdomen, performed with the patient in the supine position, are sufficient: one anteroposterior (AP) radiograph and one laterolateral (LL) radiograph with the X-ray tube parallel to the floor. The abdominal plain films should be completed with a chest radiograph (AP radiograph in the supine position).

LL Radiograph in the Supine Position (Scheme 5.1)

- Shows intestinal stasis.
- Demonstrates features of abdominal wall and bowel loops.
- Defines the relationship between intestine and abdominal wall.
- Reveals free intraperitoneal air.

AP Radiograph in the Supine Position (Scheme 5.2)

- Offers an overview of gastrointestinal abnormalities.
- Defines the relationship between intestine and abdominal wall.
- Reveals free intraperitoneal air.

Cooperative Patient

It is possible to perform the complete "basic series" in such a patient: one posteroanterior (PA) radiograph in the prone position, and one PA radiograph in the upright position are added to the supine radiographs. In the PA films, the bowel loops are near the sensitive plane and are compressed. The chest radiological study should be performed in the double projections.

PA Radiograph in the Prone Position (Scheme 5.3)

- Allows a careful and detailed analysis of bowel aspects and relationship.
- Allows visualisation of the intestinal content in a different distribution with respect to the supine position.

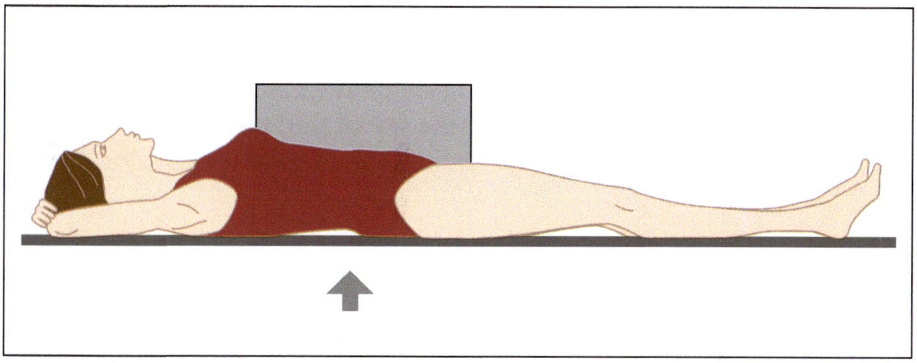

Scheme 5.1. Patient in supine decubitus: laterolateral radiograph

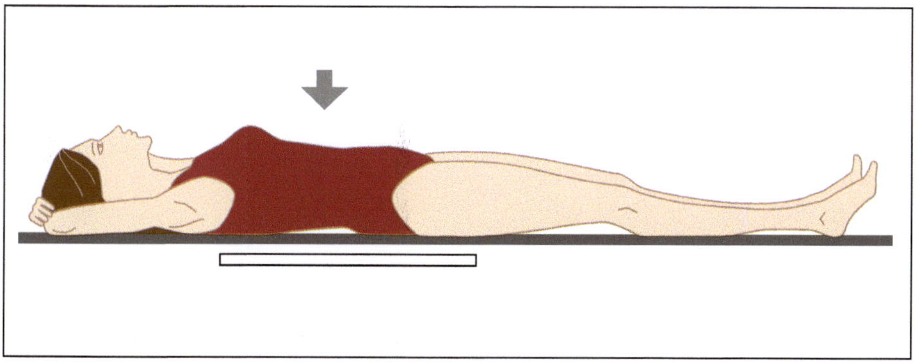

Scheme 5.2. Patient in supine decubitus: anteroposterior radiograph

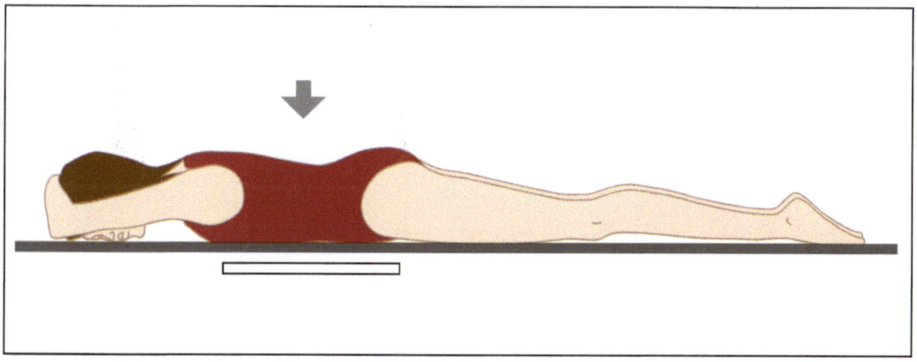

Scheme 5.3. Patient in prone decubitus: posteroanterior radiograph

PA Radiograph in the Upright Position (Scheme 5.4)

- Shifts the gaseous–liquid stasis and creates air–fluid levels.
- Allows evaluation of the entity and the site of the stasis.
- Facilitates the subphrenic disposition of free air and the pelvic location of free peritoneal fluid.

It may be useful to perform two additional radiographs, one in the left and one in the right lateral decubitus, focused to the rectal ampulla. The aim is to shift intestinal air. It is important to analyse left and right lateral decubitus. The continuity of intestinal canalisation allows the gas to reach

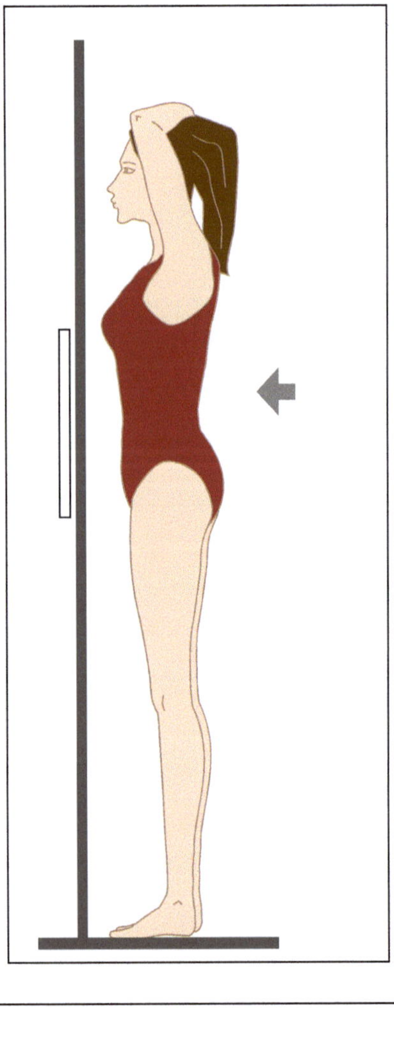

Scheme 5.4. Patient in upright position: posteroanterior radiograph

and distend the rectal ampulla. On the other hand, in the presence of an organic interruption to canalisation, the air will reach the rectal ampulla at a minimal rate and in an inhomogeneous and fragmentary manner.

In the follow-up, it is unnecessary to perform the entire "basic series": the more appropriate radiographs should be selected based on individual cases.

Acute Intestinal Behaviours

The acute intestinal behaviours indicate all variations of tone, motility, shape and location that the intestine may assume in acute pathologic conditions. Actually, the bowel loop changes its aspect, tone and motility and frequently its site. The acute intestinal behaviours may be divided into:

- Reflex spastic ileus (RSI).
- Reflex hypotonic ileus (RHI).
- Paralytic ileus (PI).
- Mechanical ileus (MI).

Each ileus has an intrinsic evolutive dynamism, which connects the different types to each other.

Reflex Spastic Ileus

RSI presents with abdominal cramps due to intense spasticity of the intestine. The radiographic findings are (Figs. 5.1–5.5):

- The marked reduction or total absence of intestinal gas in the usual sites and modes (intestinal silence): the hypertonic–spastic condition of the bowel causes the almost total absence of normal findings of intestinal gas.
- Regular or enhanced visibility of the normal abdominal features: the contracture of the abdominal musculature highlights the visibility of the parenchymal organs, and the parietal and visceral findings, such as the flank stripe, the borders of the psoas muscles and the pelvic floor.

RSI may represent the onset of acute abdomen, regardless of the underlying cause, and it may often escape radiological documentation, giving its early appearance. It may be transient, with spontaneous resolution within a few hours; however, in most cases, it develops into hypotonic ileus. Persistence of intestinal spasticity represents a cause for alarm, indicating the presence of a serious pathologic condition.

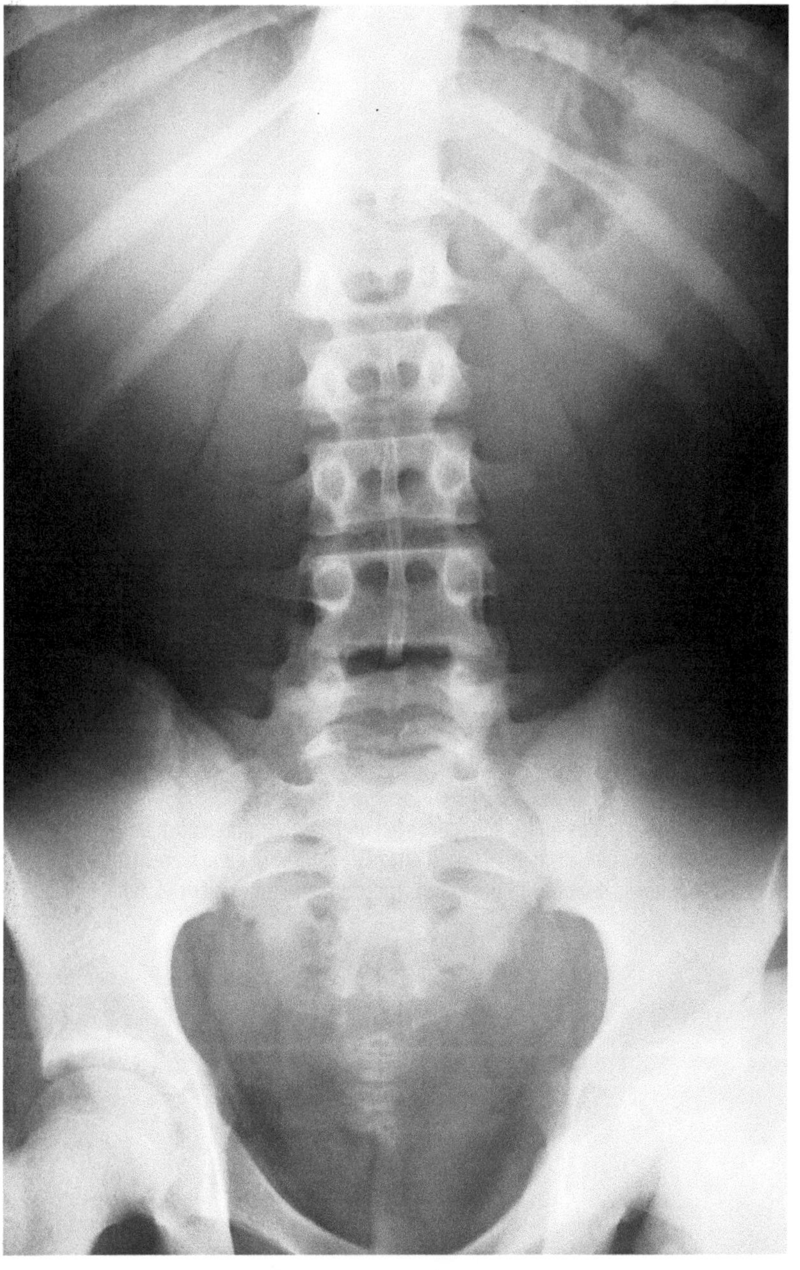

Fig. 5.1. Diffuse reflex spastic ileus by hepatic contusion. Anteroposterior supine radiograph. Complete intestinal silence, except for minimal amount of air in the gastric cavity (From Grassi R et al. (2004) Semeiotica radiografica dell'addome acuto all'esame radiologico diretto: ileo riflesso spastico, ileo riflesso ipotonico, ileo meccanico ed ileo paralitico. Radiol Med 108:56–70, reproduced with permission)

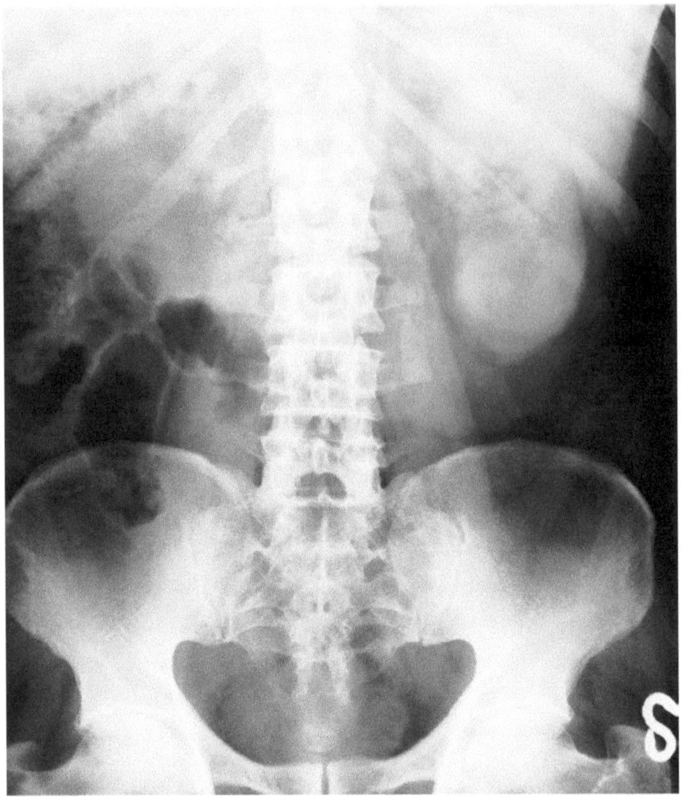

Fig. 5.2. Localised reflex spastic ileus due to left ureteral colic. Anteroposterior supine radiograph. Right abdomen shows a substantially normal aspect and placement of gas and faeces. Left abdomen shows intestinal silence and good visualisation of kidney, psoas muscle, flank stripe and pelvic floor

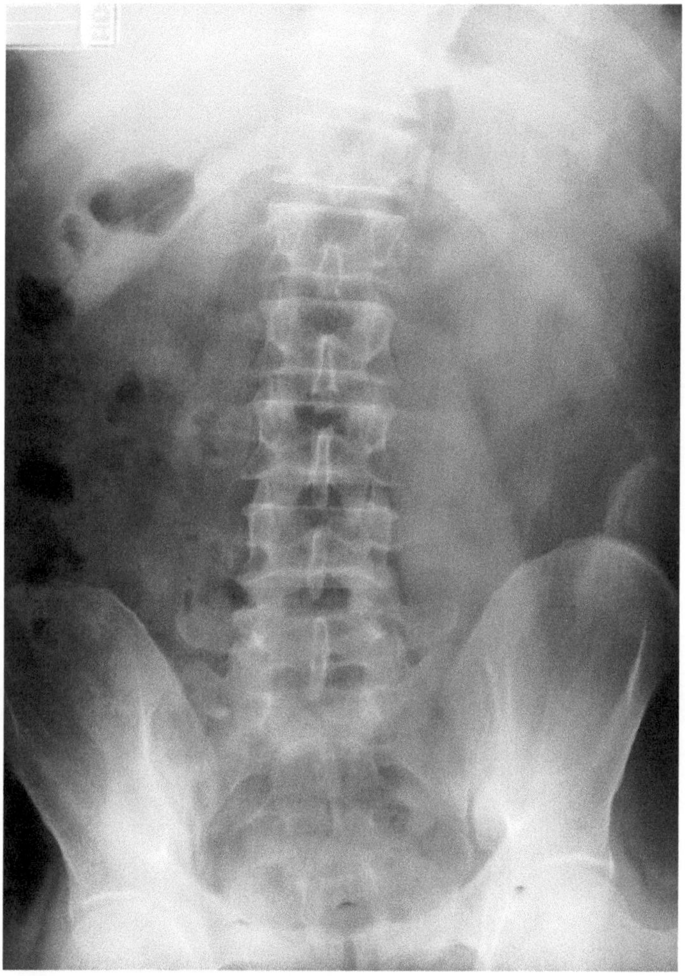

Fig. 5.3. Localised reflex spastic ileus due to left ureteral colic. Posteroanterior prone radiograph. Normal-shaped faeces in right colon. Spine in antalgic left deflected position. Absence of gas and faeces in left abdomen. Contraction of abdominal wall causes muscular wall thickening of the left flank

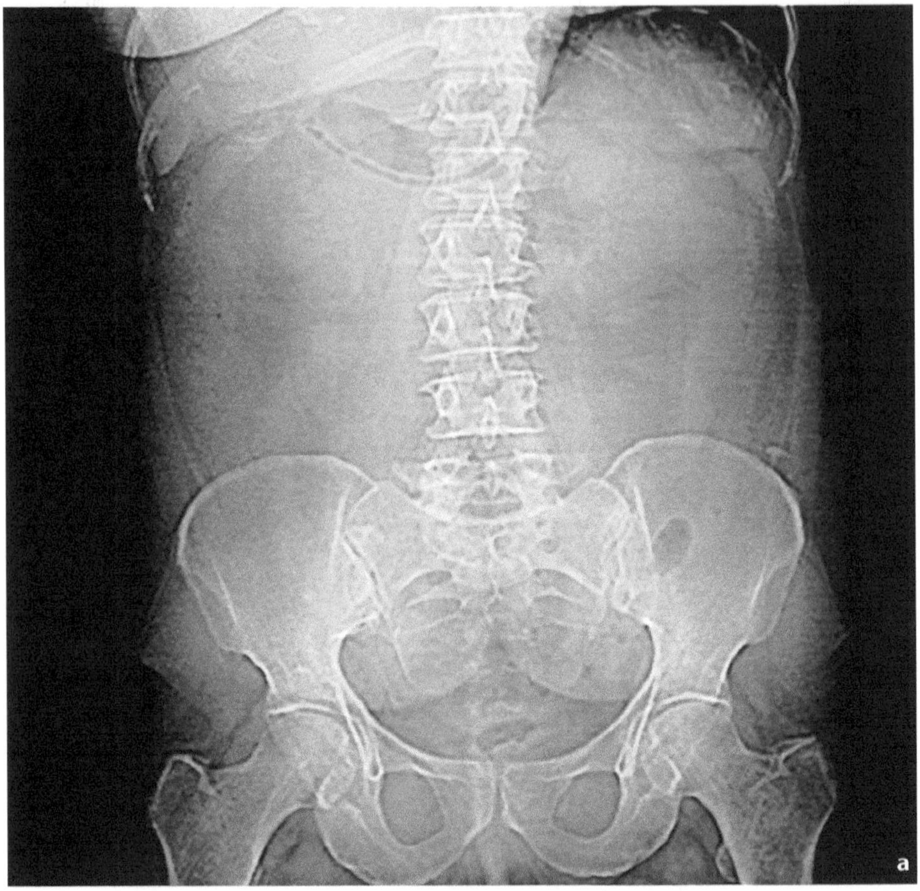

Fig. 5.4 a-c. Diffuse reflex spastic ileus due to acute appendicitis. Contrast-enhanced multidetector computed tomography (CT). **a** Anteroposterior scout view. Presence of nasogastric tube. Violent hypertonic spastic crisis of intestine causes almost complete absence of intestinal gas. **b, c** CT appearance of contracted and collapsed jejunal loops. Normal mesentery. Absence of peritoneal fluid (*cont.* →)

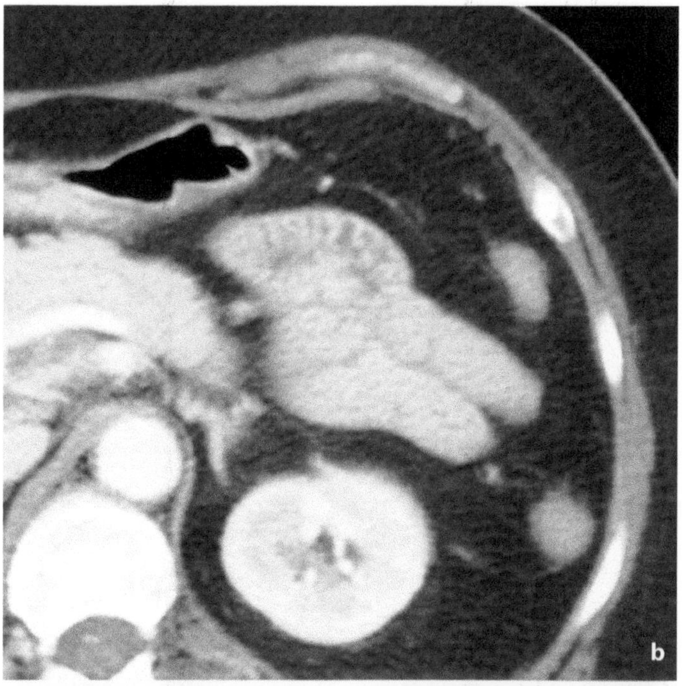
b

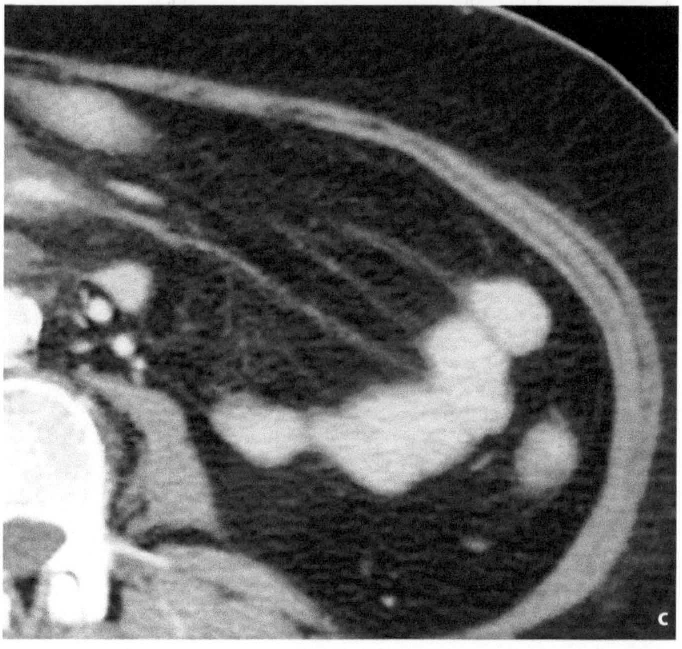
c

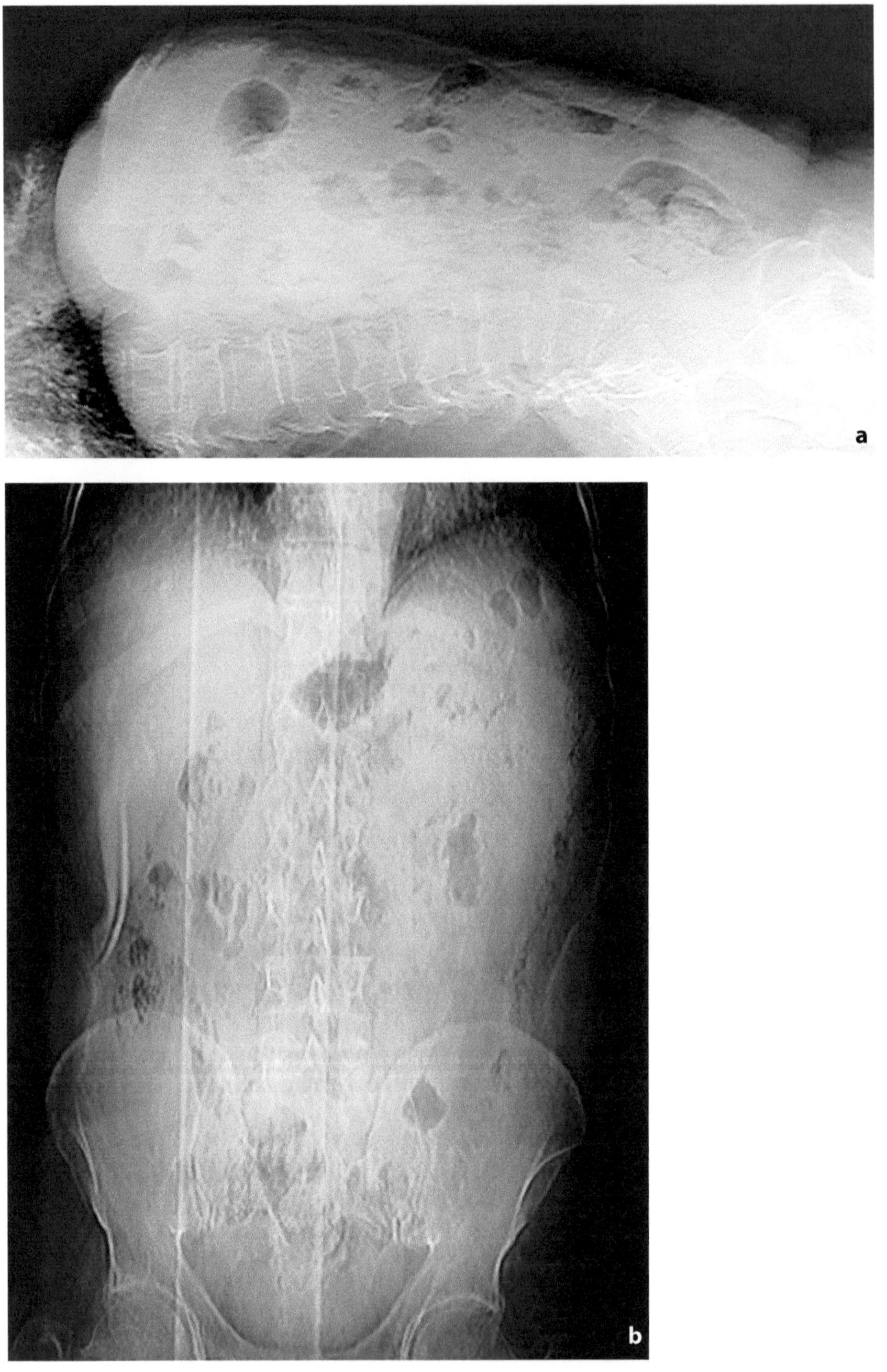

Fig. 5.5 a-d. Evolution of reflex spastic ileus. Multifocal spastic ileus following trauma with multiple lumbar vertebral fractures. **a, b** Frontal and lateral scout views. Poor, inhomogeneous and multisegmental distribution of intestinal gaseous content. Absence of fluid levels. Absence of abdominal distension. (*cont.* →)

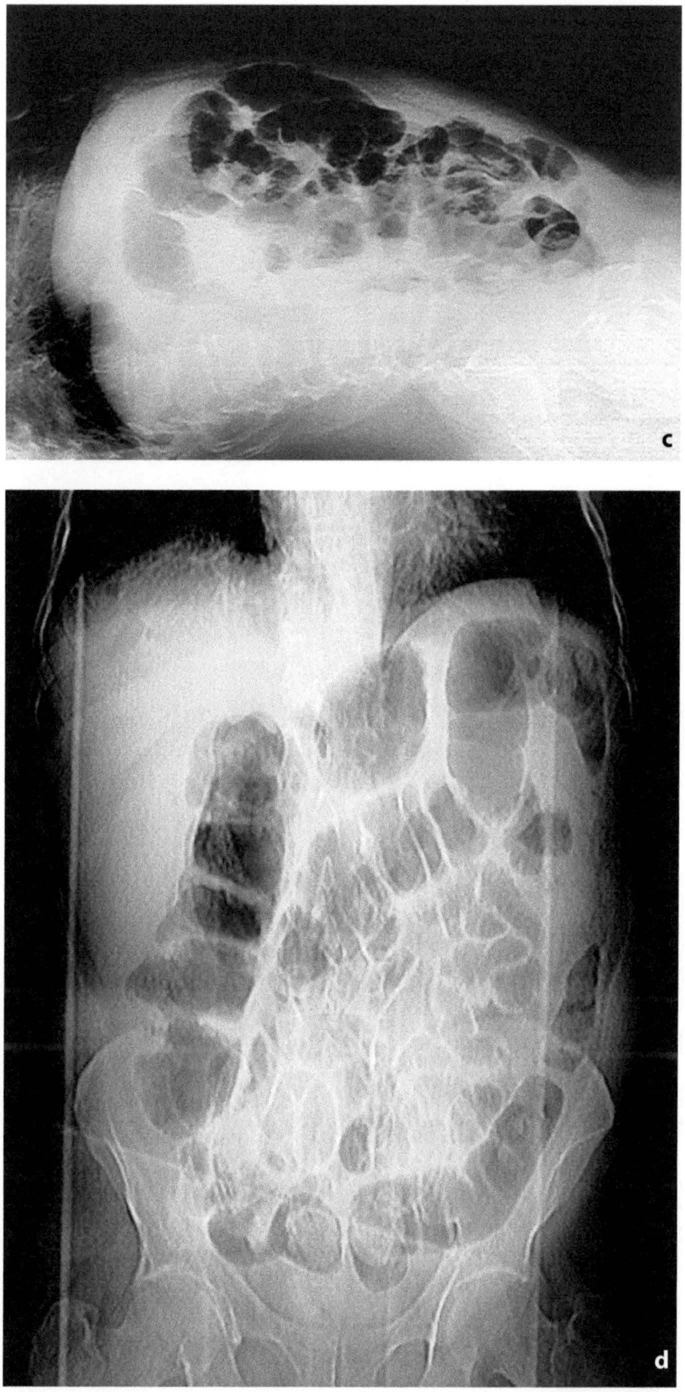

c, d Follow-up at 24 h. Frontal and lateral scout views. Hypertonic spastic reaction has disappeared. Subsequent tone reduction determined a clinical and radiological picture of abdominal and intestinal distension. Diffuse and homogeneous, but moderate, dilatation of small and large bowel. Exclusively gaseous stasis. Spastic ileus has progresses to hypotonic ileus

Reflex Hypotonic Ileus

When hypertonic–spastic reaction ends, the bowel loop relaxes and the tone decreases, with a clinical picture of intestinal distension (Figs. 5.6–5.8). RHI is characterised by:

- homogeneous reduction of tone;
- gaseous stasis;
- absence of fluid levels;
- moderate distension;
- thin walls;
- slight or absent valvulae conniventes;
- bowel loops crowded in a geometric or mosaic pattern.

RHI may be transient, and its progressive resolution is revealed by the appearance of different intestinal tone and motility abnormalities. RHI deterioration is documented by the appearance of fluid stasis, which demonstrates the evolution into a different and more serious ileus of the paralytic variety. Gaseous stasis forms when tone decreases. Liquid stasis forms only when kinesis decreases.

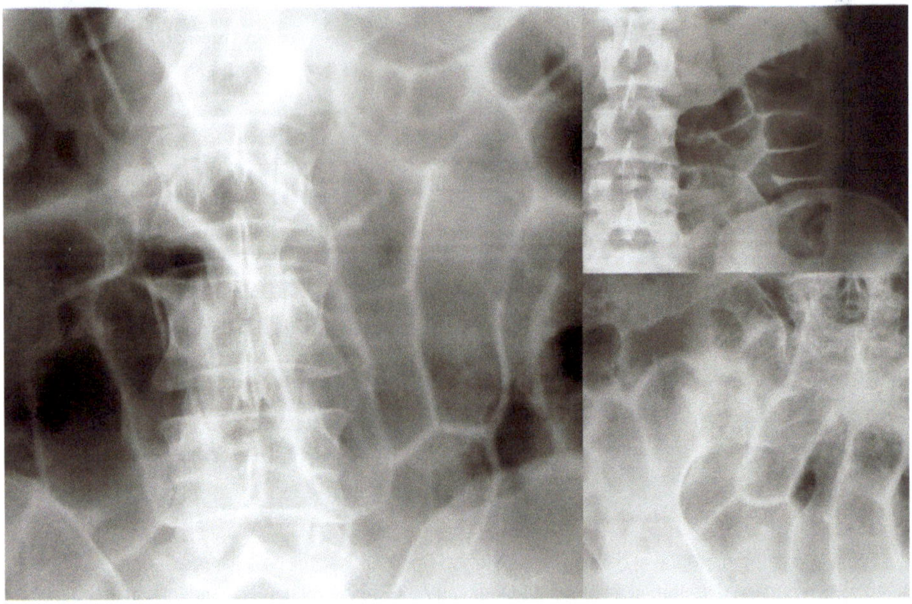

Fig. 5.6. Reflex hypotonic ileus. Loop image. Anteroposterior supine radiographs of three patients. Moderate small-bowel distension. Thin walls and almost absent valvulae conniventes. Characteristic crowding of loops, with geometric mosaic pattern. (From Grassi R et al. (2004) Semeiotica radiografica dell'addome acuto all'esame radiologico diretto: ileo riflesso spastico, ileo riflesso ipotonico, ileo meccanico ed ileo paralitico. Radiol Med 108:56–70, reproduced with permission)

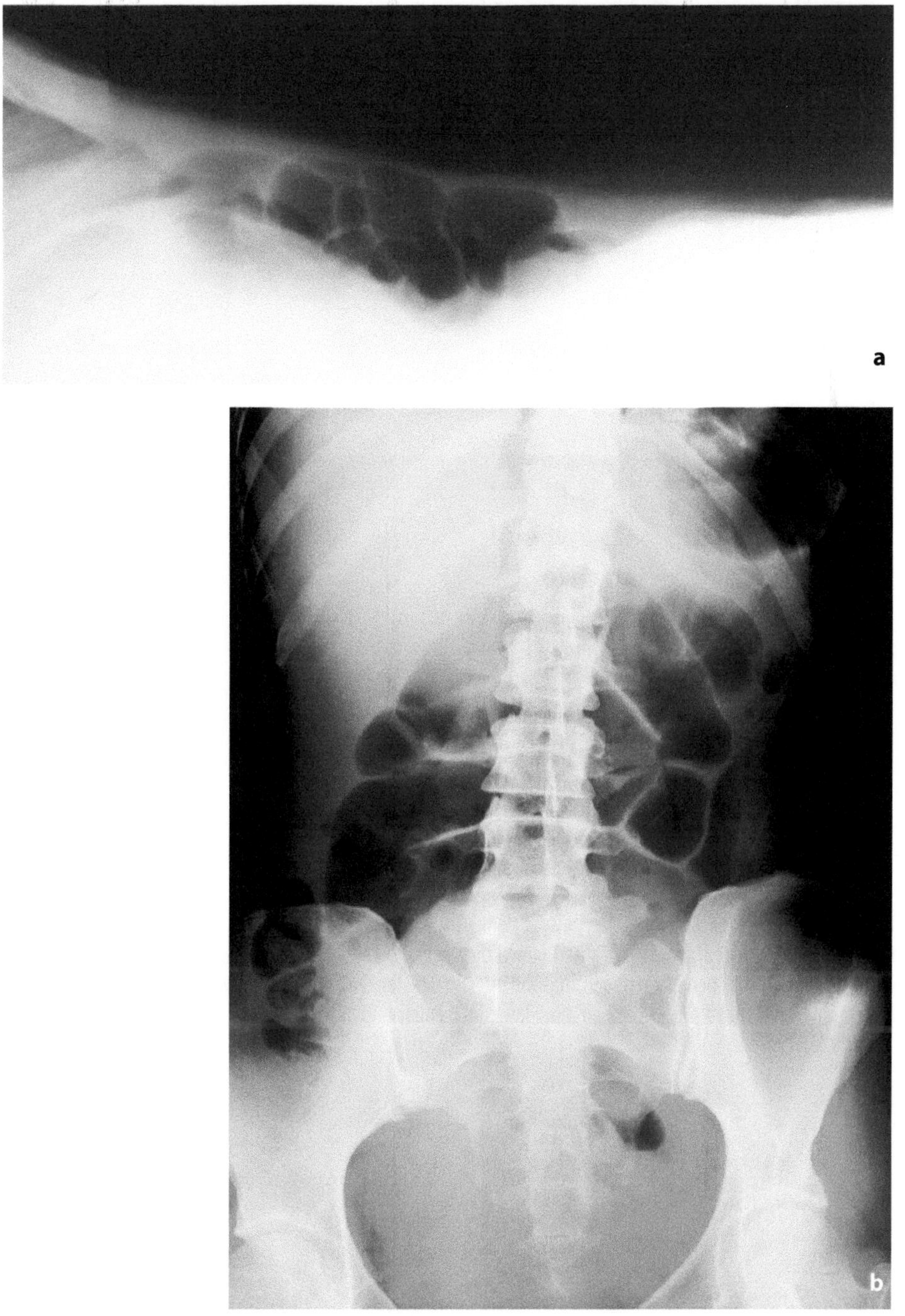

Fig. 5.7 a, b. Localised reflex hypotonic ileus due to heroine overdose. **a, b** Laterolateral supine radiograph. Anteroposterior supine radiograph. Exclusively gaseous stasis. Distension limited to some small-bowel loops. Colic frame barely detectable. In mid left abdomen, a characteristic mosaic pattern of loops is evident

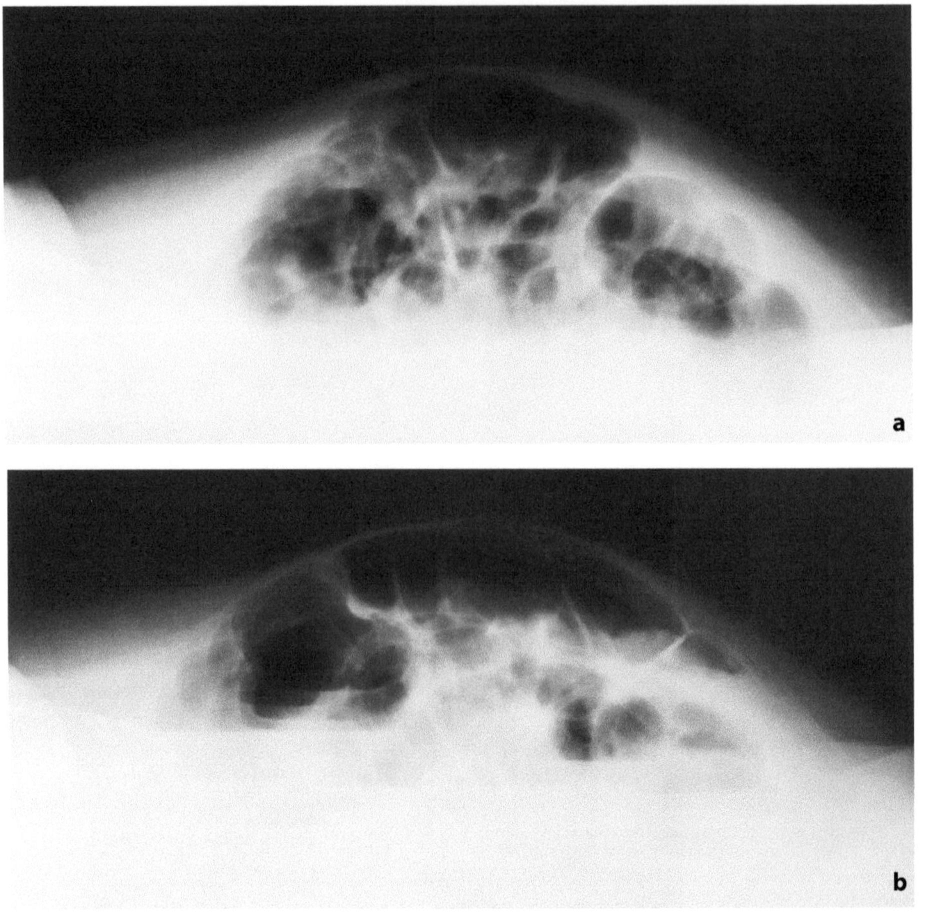

Fig. 5.8 a-d. Evolution of reflex hypotonic ileus (RHI). Serious cardiac and circulatory failure. **a** Laterolateral (LL) supine radiograph. Gaseous small-bowel distension. **b** Follow-up at 24 h. LL supine radiograph. Evidence of liquid stasis. Increasing abdominal and intestinal distension with colon involvement. RHI has changed into paralytic ileus with presence of air-fluid levels. **c, d** Follow-up at 48 h. (*cont.* →)

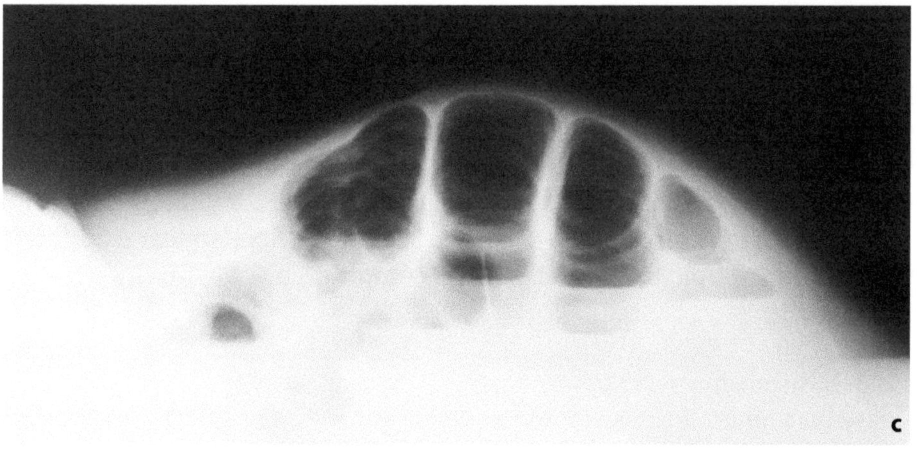

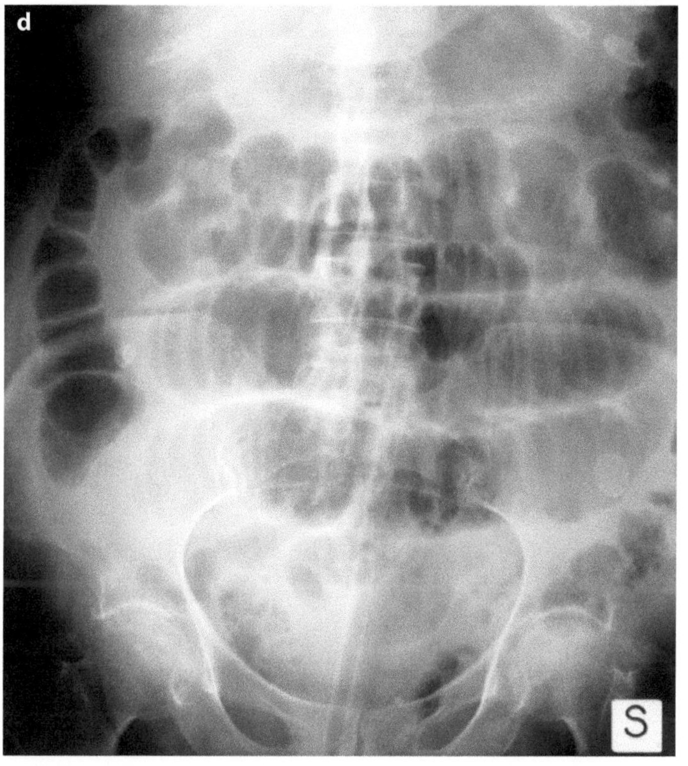

c LL supine radiograph. Further increase of loop diameter and liquid stasis. Tone and motility reduction reaches complete paralysis. **d** Anteroposterior supine radiograph. Frontal panoramic view confirms small- and large-bowel distension. Gastric involvement indicates a serious condition. Tone and motility reduction causes horizontal distribution of some jejunal loops. A rectal catheter has been introduced to reduce abdominal and intestinal distension. The patient died within a few hours

Paralytic Ileus

PI, or dynamic ileus, represents an acute functional abnormality of canalisation due to reduction of intestinal tone and motility. In PI, continuity of the intestinal lumen is maintained. It may involve primarily or exclusively the small bowel, either the large bowel, or both (Figs. 5.9–5.14). Gastric involvement is indicative of seriousness. PI has multiple appearances and, therefore, its radiological description is complex. The only findings always present are:

- bowel distension;
- gaseous and liquid stasis;
- reduction of tone and motility.

In the follow-up, resolution of PI is revealed by:

- reduction of bowel-loop diameter;
- reduction of liquid stasis;
- restoration of intestinal tone and motility.

Deterioration of PI is characterised by:

- increase of bowel-loop diameter;
- increase of liquid stasis;
- progressive reduction of tone and motility up to paralysis.

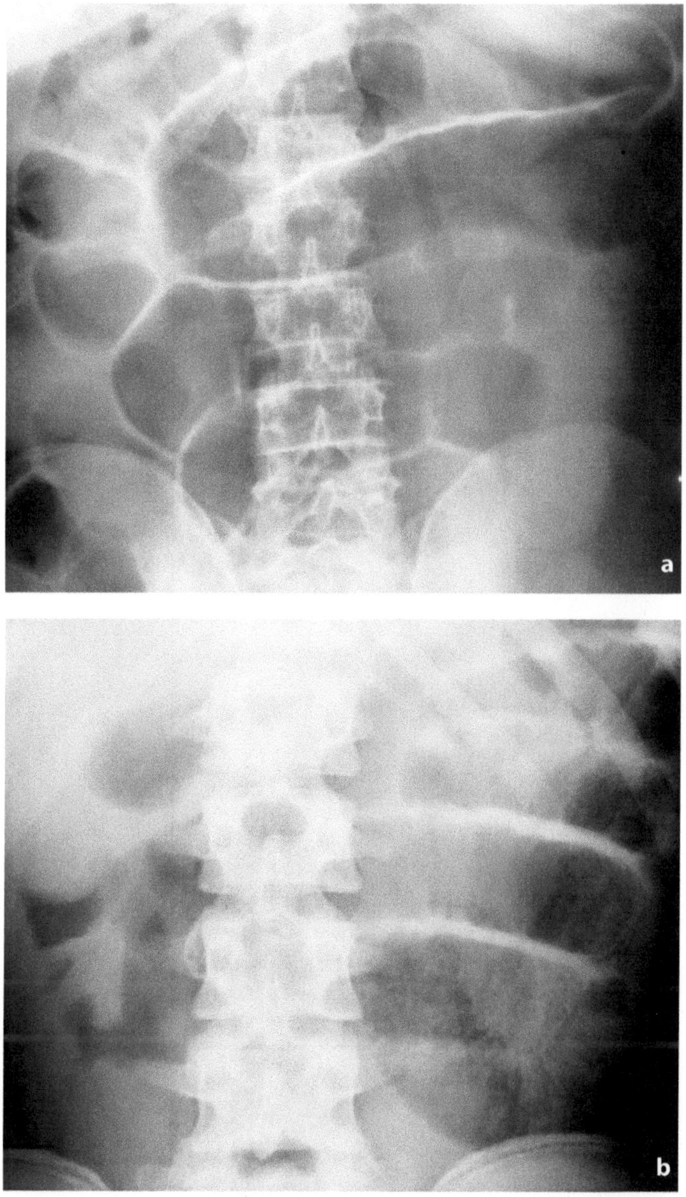

Fig. 5.9 a, b. Paralytic ileus. Loop image. **a, b** Anteroposterior supine radiographs of two patients who showed air–liquid levels in upright radiographs (not shown). **a** Drug overdose for attempted suicide. Significant tone and motility reduction causes a rectilinear disposition of small-bowel loops. Focal, loop crowding with geometric pattern. **b** Peritonitis due to complicated acute appendicitis. Increase of abdomen opacity by conspicuous peritoneal fluid. Dilated jejunal loops tend towards a horizontal distribution. Poorly visualised valvulae conniventes

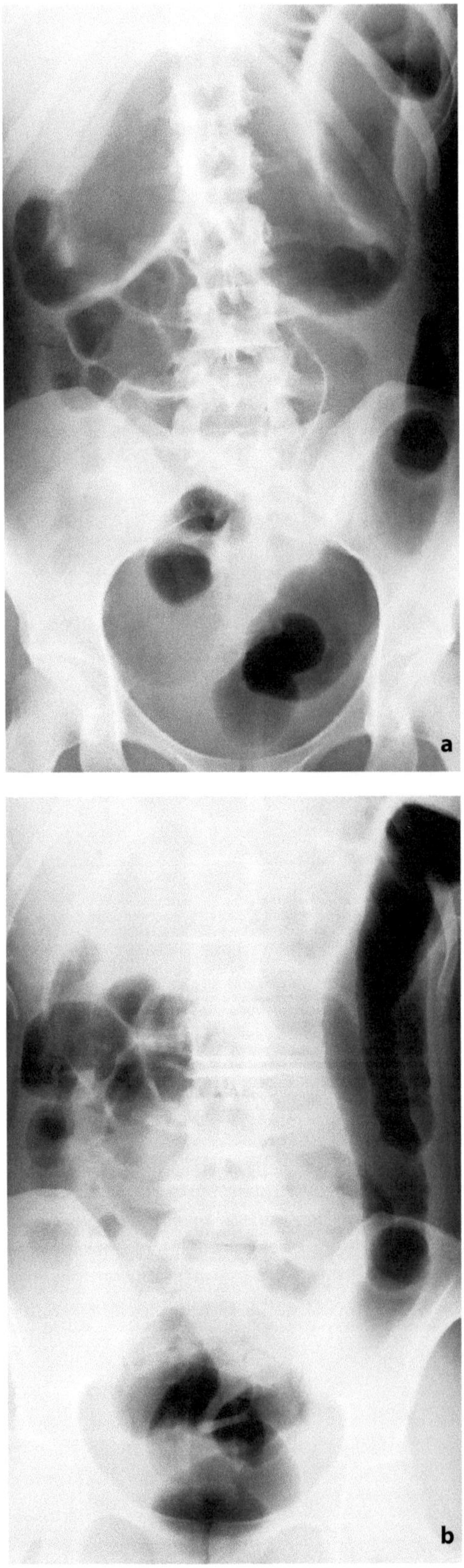

Fig. 5.10 a, b. Paralytic ileus. Anaesthetic drug overdose. **a** Anteroposterior supine radiograph. **b** Posteroanterior prone radiograph. Significant distension of small and large bowel. Continuity of intestinal canalisation allows gas to move freely with change of patient's position: rectal ampulla well distended in the prone position

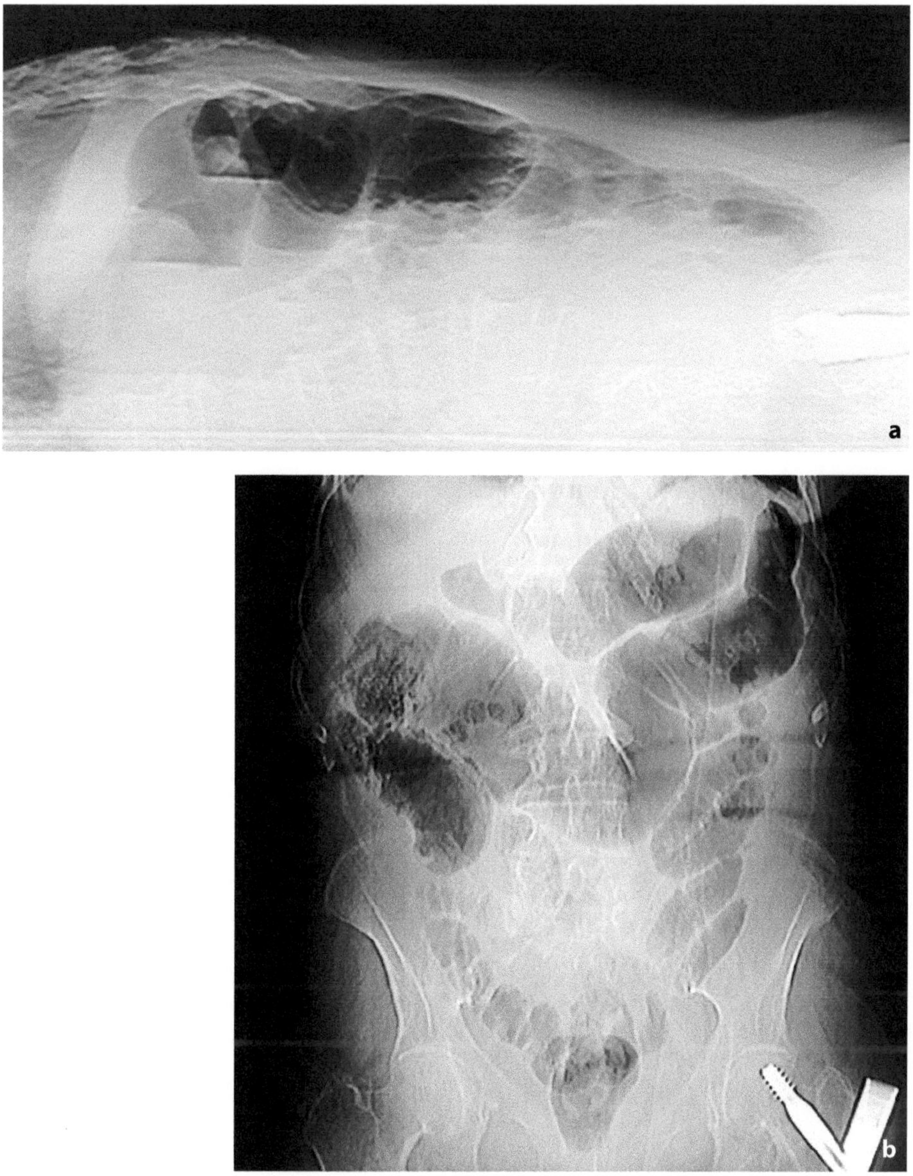

Fig. 5.11 a, b. Paralytic ileus by severe cerebral ischaemia. **a** Laterolateral supine radiograph. Mixed gastrointestinal stasis. **b** Anteroposterior supine radiograph. Panoramic radiographs allow visualisation of the stasis in the distended viscera: stomach, small bowel, colon, rectum

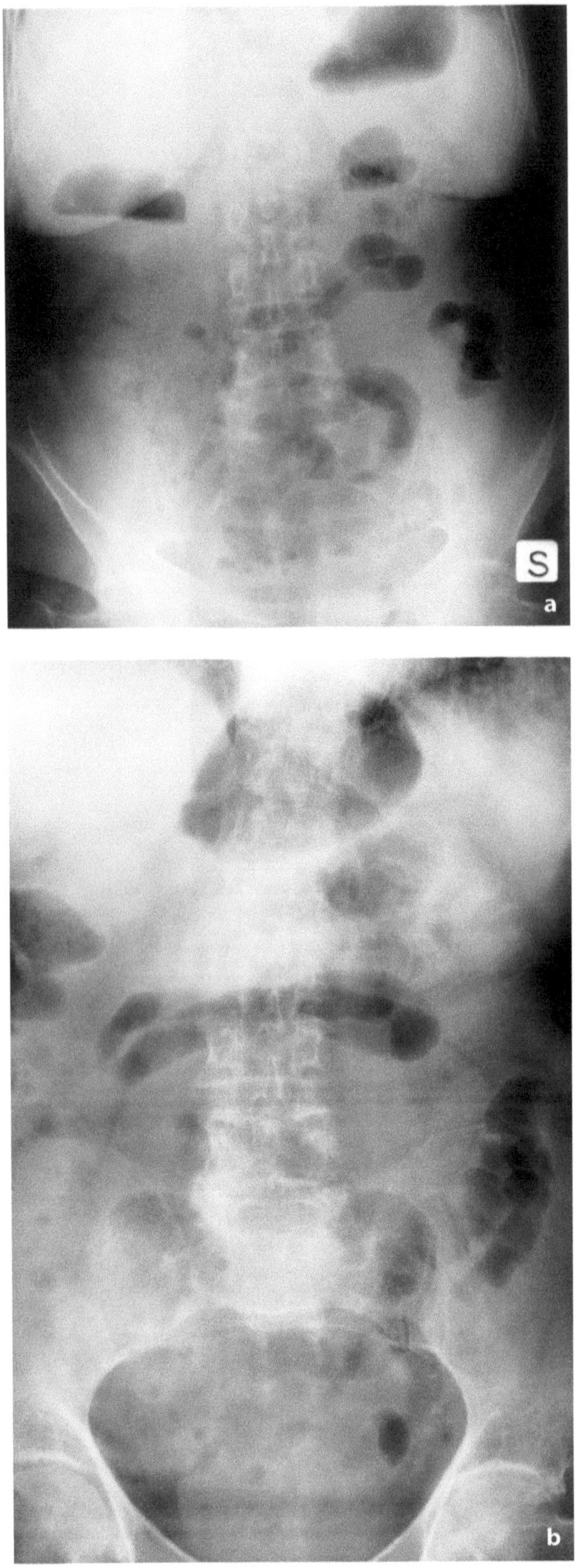

Fig. 5.12 a,b. Paralytic ileus. Massive arterial small-bowel infarction. **a** Posteroanterior upright radiograph. **b** Supine anteroposterior radiograph. Moderate small-bowel distension with gas-liquid stasis. Gastric and right colon ectasia. In mid abdomen, two small-bowel loops tend to the horizontal distribution. Gas-containing loops show thin walls without valvulae conniventes

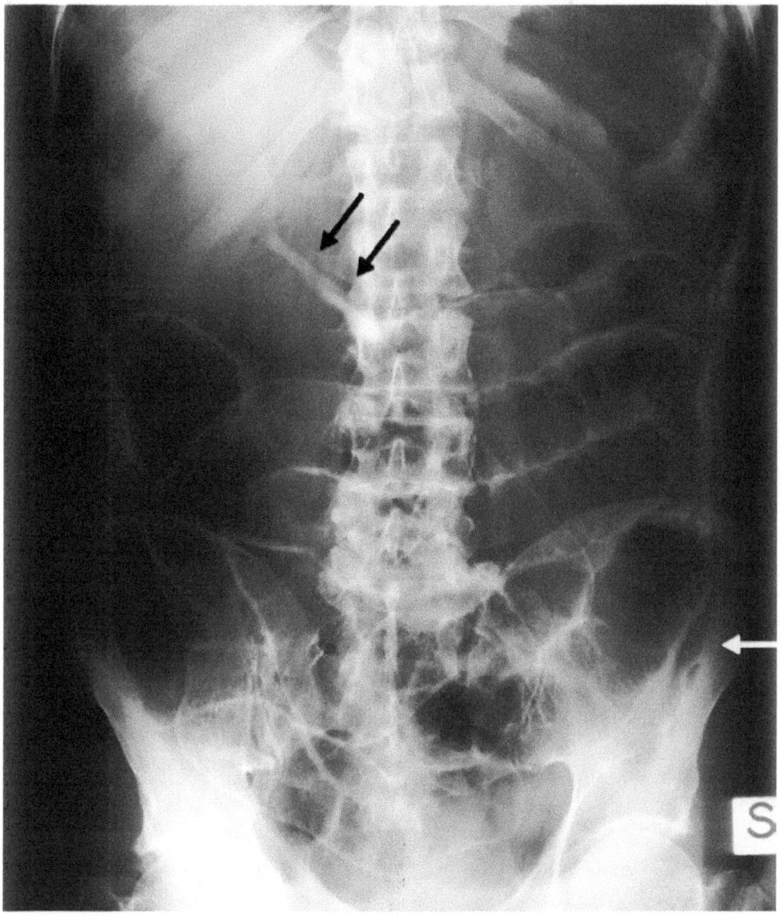

Fig. 5.13. Paralytic ileus. Peritonitis due to perforated sigmoid colon diverticulum with free peritoneal and retroperitoneal air. Anteroposterior supine radiograph. Free peritoneal air is confirmed by the presence of Rigler's sign, "bright liver" and presence of the round ligament (*black arrows*). Free retroperitoneal air is demonstrated by presence of gas in the left posterior pararenal space (*white arrow*). Massive gaseous small-bowel distension. Drastic tone reduction causes tendency of loops to a horizontal distribution. Gas-containing bowel shows thin walls and incomplete valvulae conniventes

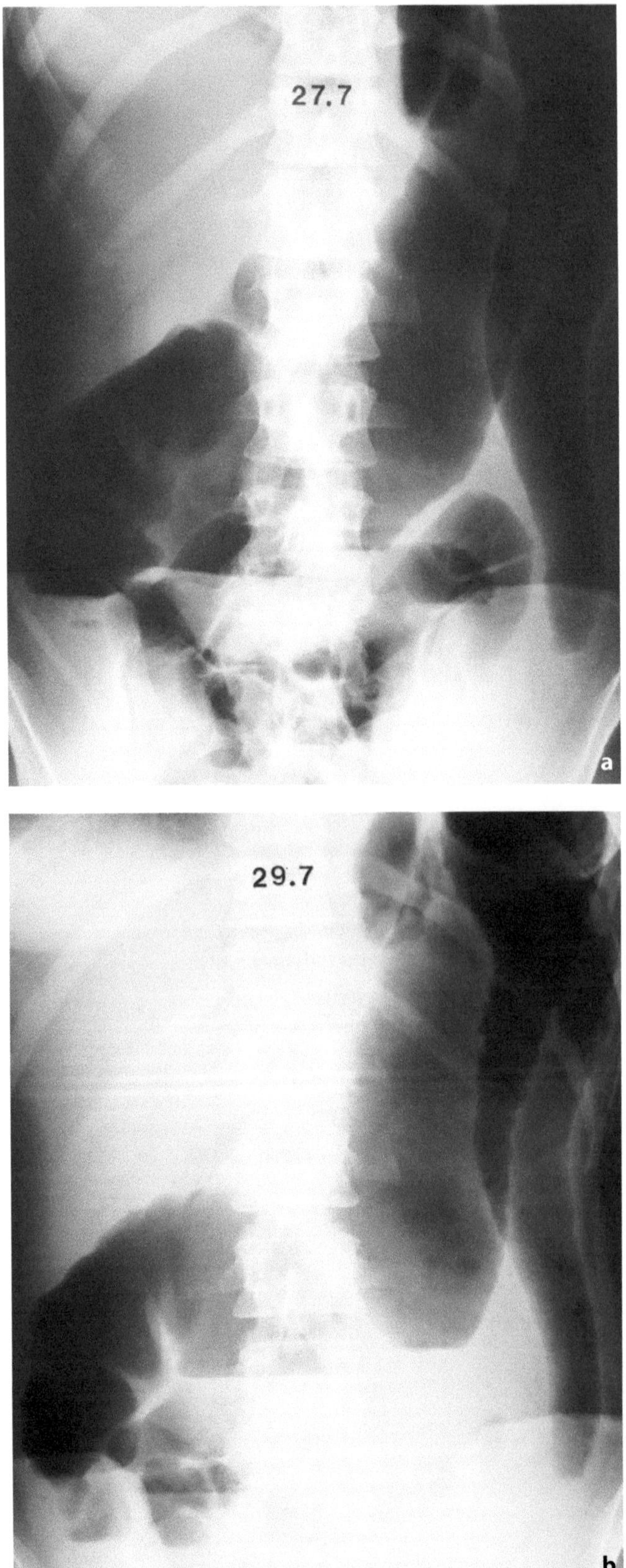

Fig. 5.14 a-e. Evolution of paralytic ileus (PI). Toxic megacolon in ulcerative colitis. Posteroanterior upright radiographs. **a** Significant colon distension is evident. Gas–liquid stasis, with a clear prevalence of gaseous component. Functional rebound of small bowel by metabolic toxin accumulation. **b** 2 days later, there is an increase in colic distension and liquid stasis due to PI worsening. (*cont.* →)

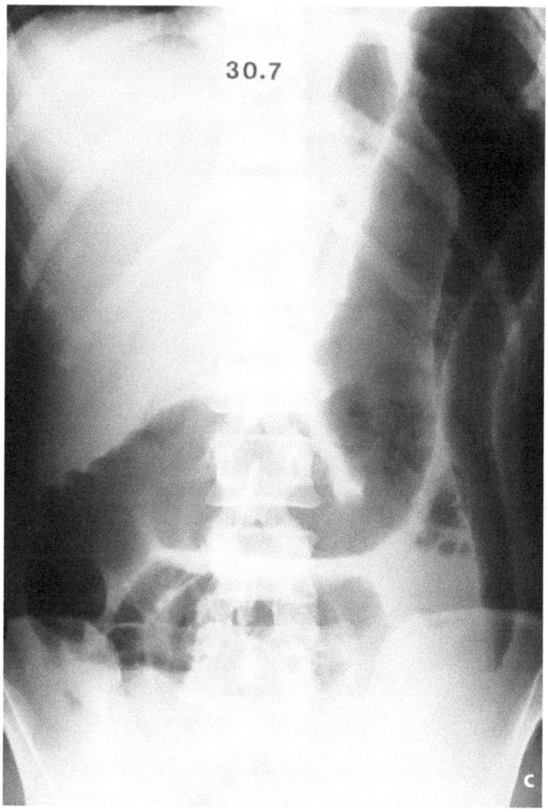

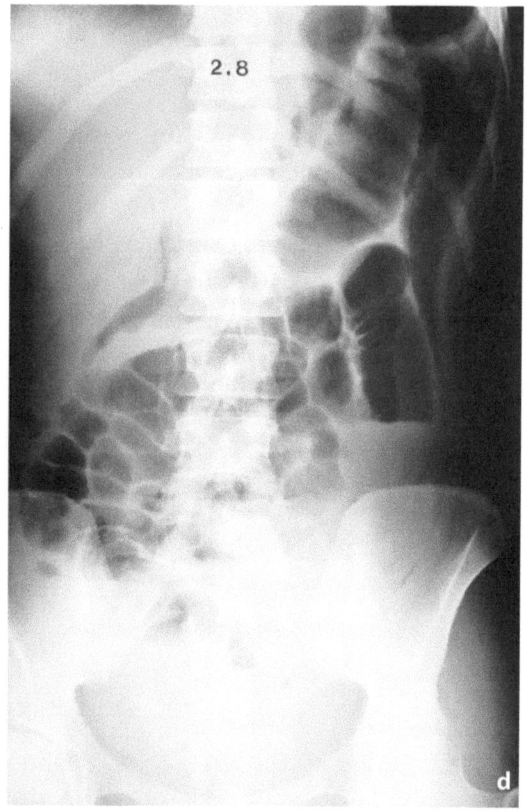

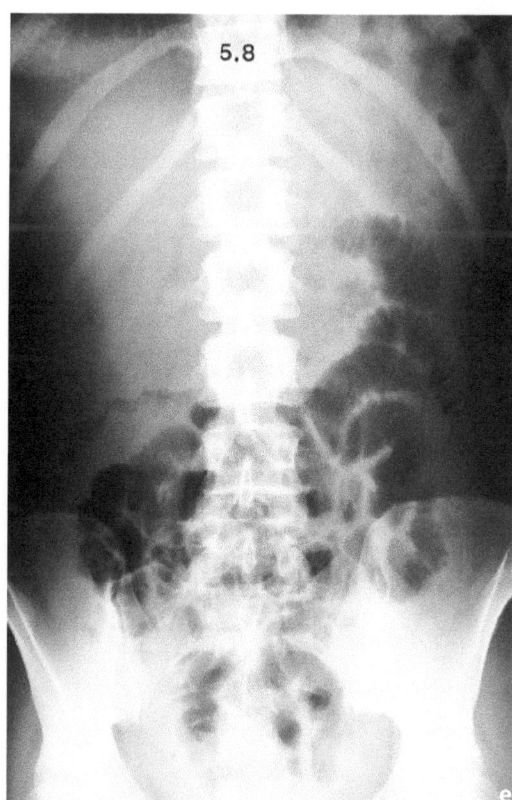

c 24 h later, there is moderate regression of PI, with reduction of colon diameter and liquid stasis. **d** 8 days later, there is further improvement with clear reduction of colon diameter and almost complete disappearance of liquid stasis. Moderate small-bowel distension with loop crowding in mosaic pattern is apparent. PI in regression has changed into hypotonic ileus. Presence of nasogastric tube. **e** 3 days later, colonic gaseous dilatation has resolved. Progressive resolution of hypotonic ileus is revealed by the appearance of intestinal tone and motility changes. Presence of nasogastric tube

Mechanical Ileus

MI is characterised by interruption of continuity of the intestinal lumen, with acute changes in canalisation (Figs. 5.15–5.20). The obstructive leading point causes an increase in intraluminal tension of the proximal loops. Loops distal to the site of obstruction show progressive collapse. Intestinal stasis is always of the mixed variety, gaseous and liquid. In simple MI, the walls are regular and thin. At the jejunum, thin valvulae conniventes with an elegant circular design with crowded and forced attitude appear rapidly, representing the final attempt of intestinal tone and motility to exceed the mechanical obstacle.

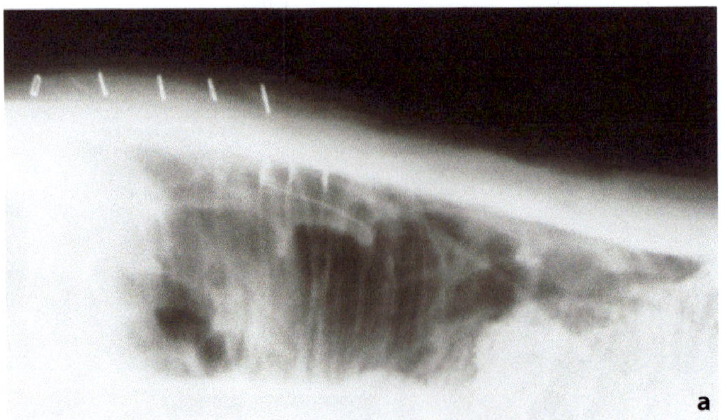

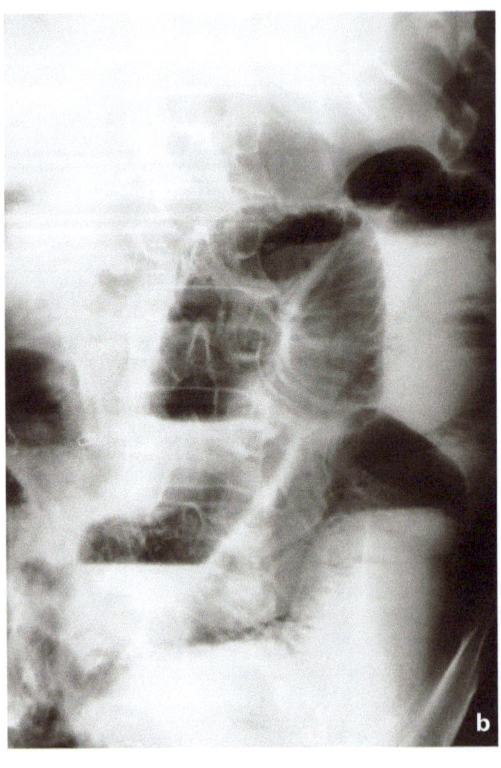

Fig. 5.15 a,b. Small-bowel obstruction due to fibrin in postoperative period. **a** Laterolateral supine radiograph and **b** posteroanterior upright radiograph. Distension of the first jejunal loops with air-fluid levels. Thin valvulae conniventes, with elegant, complete circular design. Presence of metallic clips

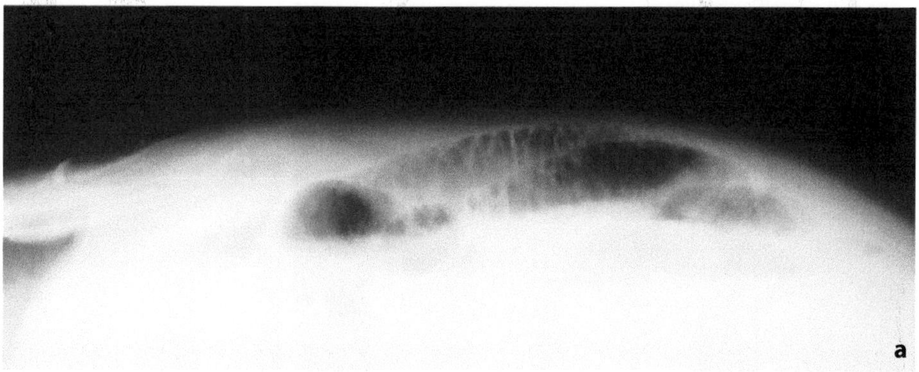

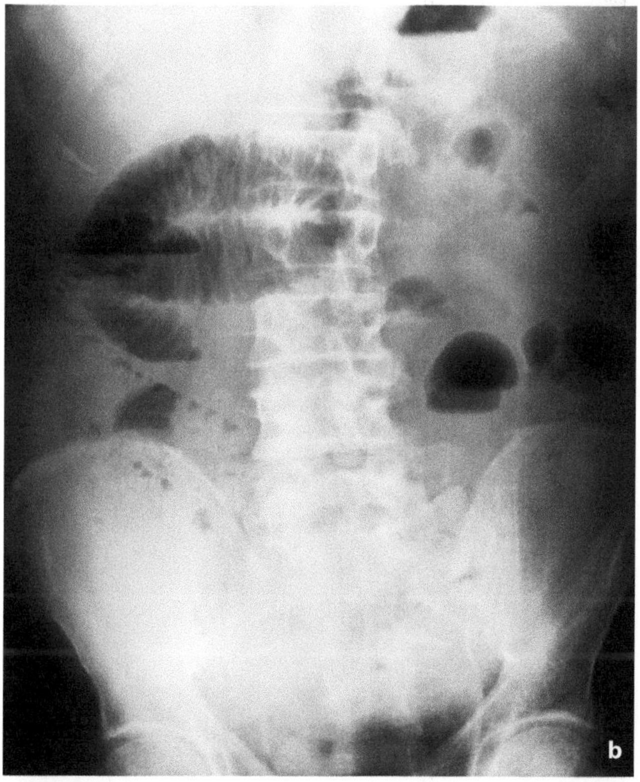

Fig. 5.16 a-f. Small-bowel obstruction. Sonographic and radiographic integration. **a-d** "Basic series" radiographs. Ileal-jejunal distension. Scantly detectable colic frame. Gas-liquid stasis. Numerous and forced valvulae conniventes. Anomalous location of jejunum on the right and of the ileum on the left side of the abdomen raises the suspicion of small-bowel volvulus. Gas-containing loops show regular and thin walls. It is impossible to express a morphological and diagnostic judgement regarding opaque liquid-containing loops in the lower abdomen. Fortunately, liquid serves as an acoustic window, and therefore allows integration between sonography and plain film. (*cont.* →)

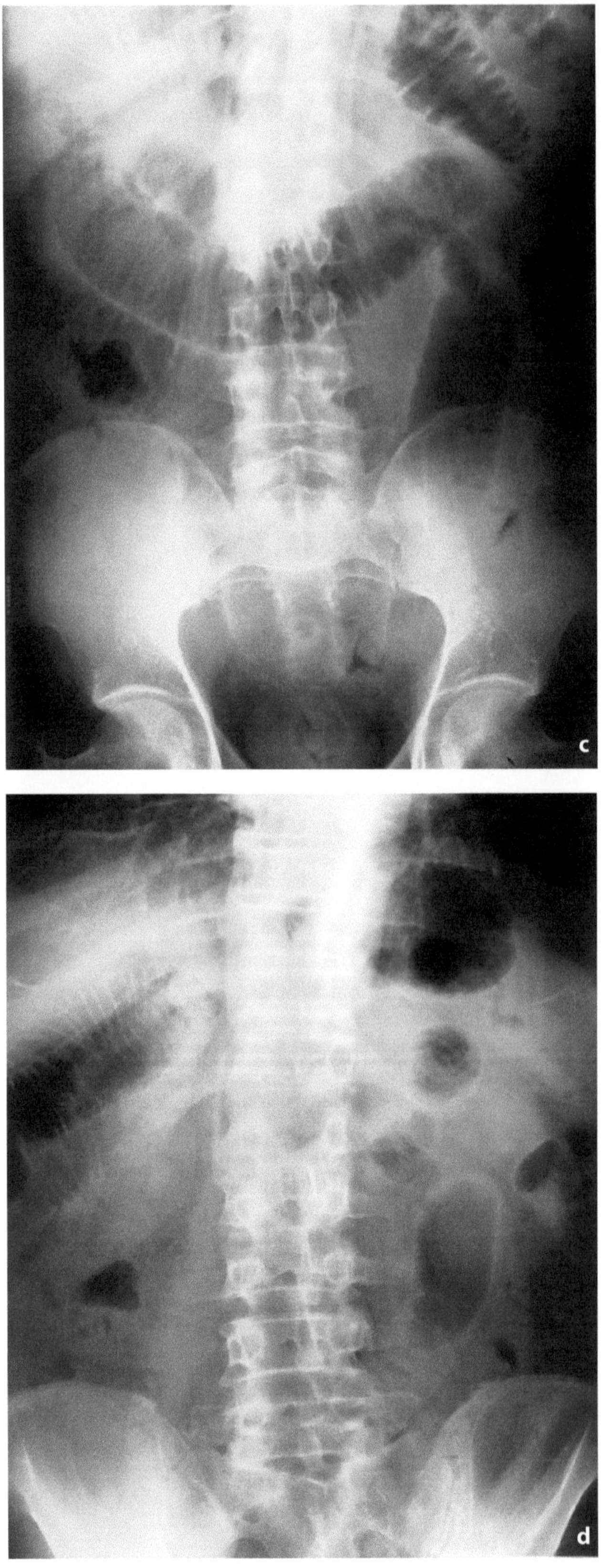

(cont. →)

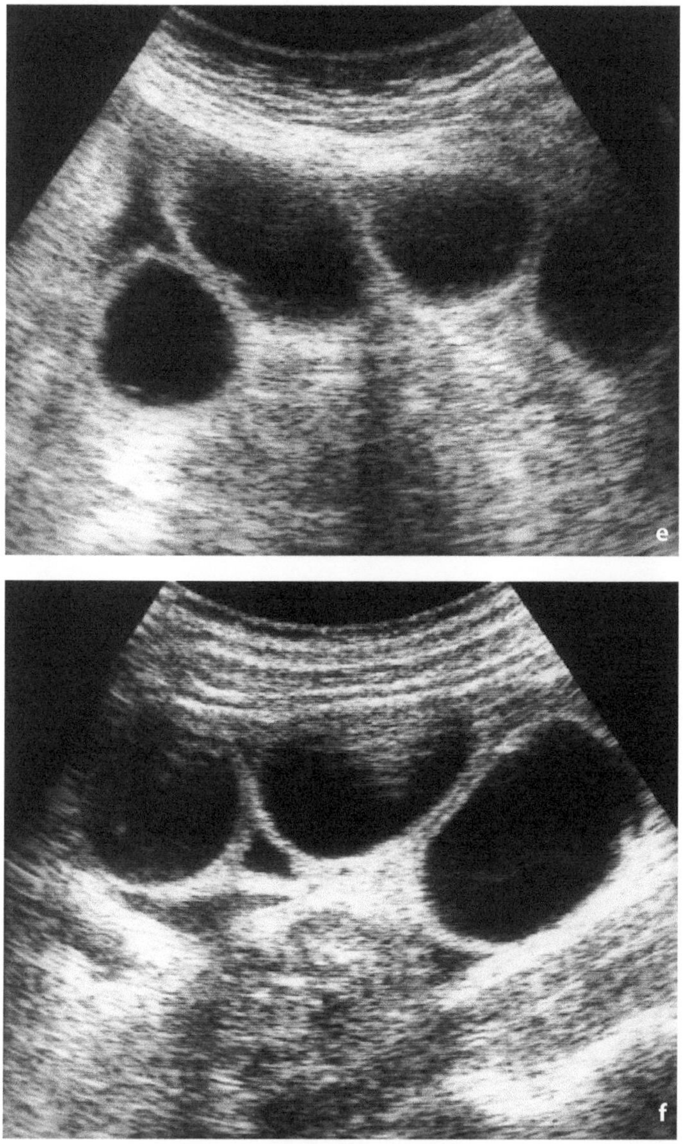

e, f Sonography. Distended ileal loops with liquid content and thin walls. Flattened valvulae conniventes due to extreme intraluminal tension. Presence of free peritoneal fluid (tanga sign). Surgery revealed subtotal small-bowel volvulus by adhesional band. (Fig. 5.16e from Grassi R et al. (2004) The relevance of free fluid between intestinal loops detected by sonography in the clinical assessment of small bowel obstruction in adults. Eur J Radiol 50:5–14, reproduced with permission)

In the follow-up, MI regression is shown by:

- reduction of liquid stasis;
- incomplete valvulae conniventes, with a less crowded and forced attitude;
- progressive reappearance of gas in the distal bowel;
- tone and motility changes.

MI worsening is characterised by:

- increase in bowel-loop diameter;
- increase in liquid stasis;
- increasingly stretched and thinned walls;
- progressive distal bowel collapse;
- tone and motility changes;
- possible development into complicated MI.

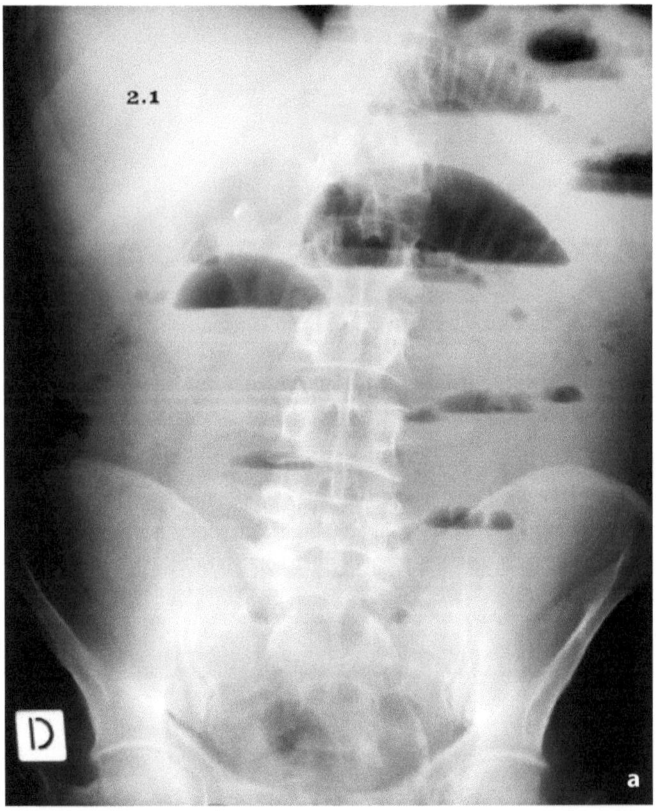

Fig. 5.17 a-c. Small-bowel obstruction regression due to a large meal. Posteroanterior upright radiographs. **a** Ileal–jejunal distension. Gas–liquid stasis with prevalence of liquid component. Forced valvulae conniventes. Absence of colic frame. (*cont.* →)

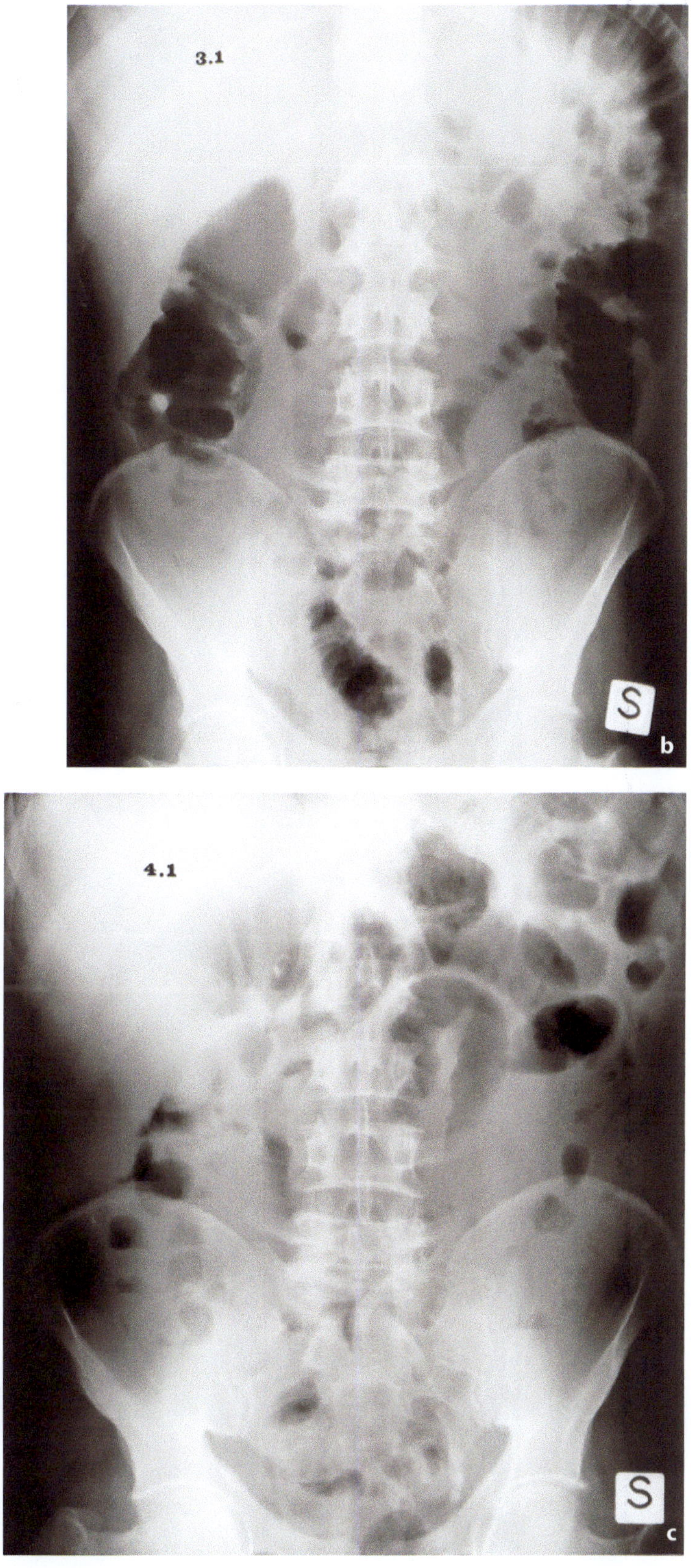

b Follow-up at 24 h. Clear reduction of small-bowel diameter and almost complete disappearance of liquid stasis. Initial gaseous replacement of large bowel. Presence of nasogastric tube. **c** Follow-up at 48 h. Liquid stasis disappearance, gaseous stasis reduction, loop diameter decrease. Progressive gaseous replacement of large bowel and presence of faeces in right colon. Tone and motility changes of small bowel persist. (From Grassi R et al. (2004) Semeiotica radiografica dell'addome acuto all'esame radiologico diretto: ileo riflesso spastico, ileo riflesso ipotonico, ileo meccanico ed ileo paralitico. Radiol Med 108:56–70, reproduced with permission)

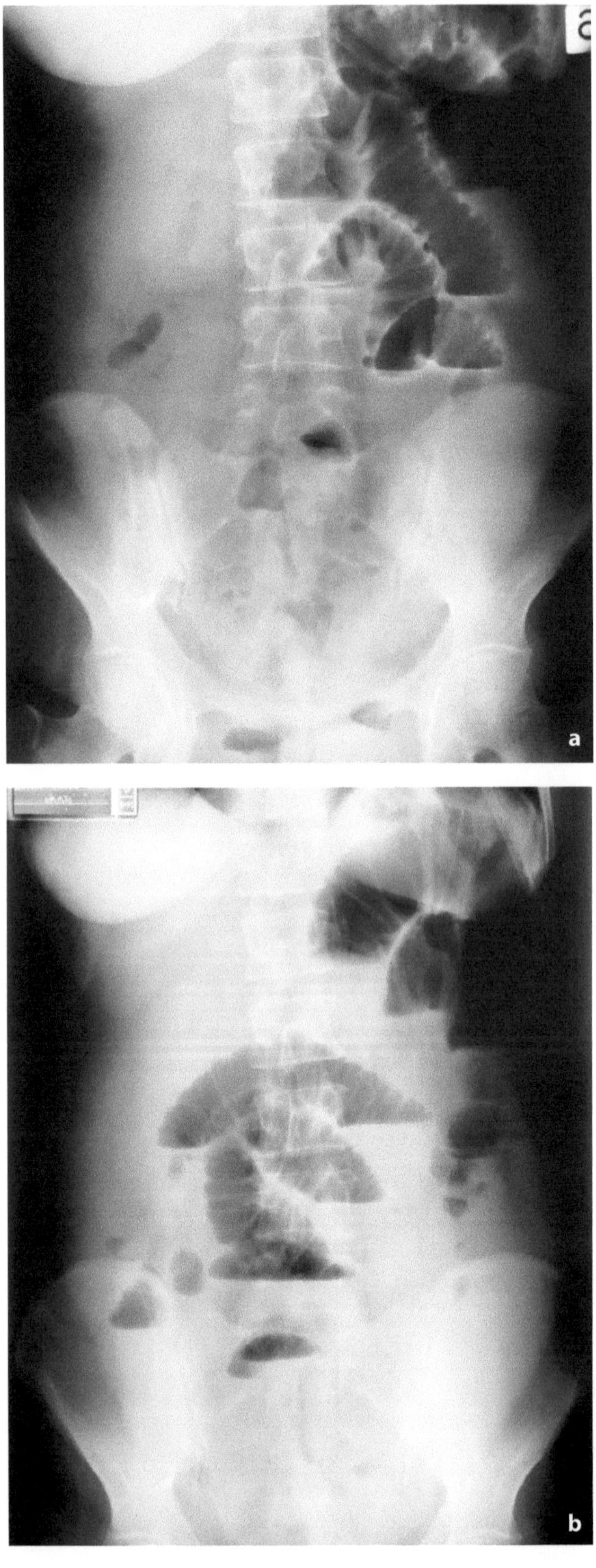

(cont. →)

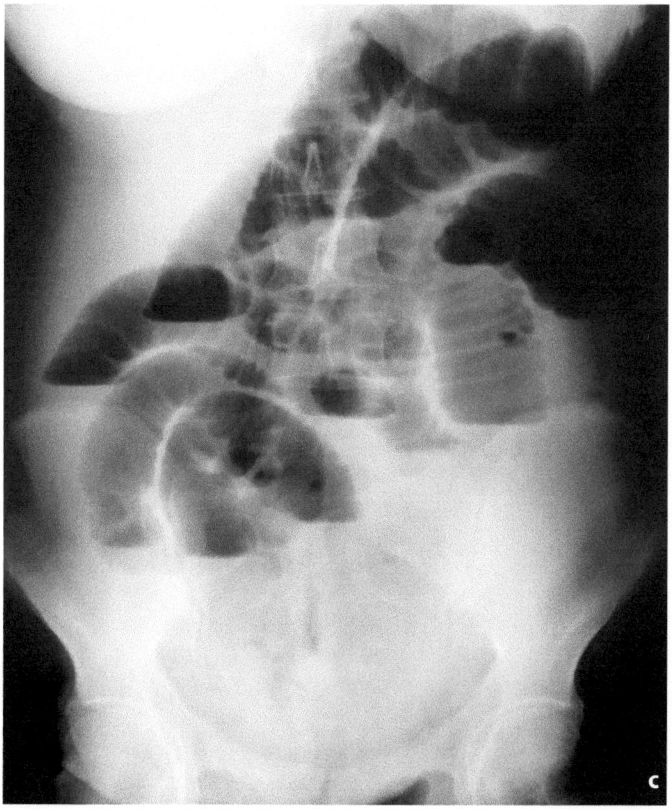

Fig. 5.18 a-c. Small-bowel obstruction (SBO) worsening. Postoperative period. Posteroanterior upright radiographs. **a** Moderate ileal–jejunal distension. Colic frame is not represented. Balanced gas–liquid stasis. Present but incomplete valvulae conniventes. **b** Follow-up at 24 h. Increase of loop diameter with imposing liquid stasis. Valvulae conniventes, with elegant complete circular design. Increase of intraluminal stasis. Radiological findings of SBO worsening. **c** Follow-up at 48 h. Abnormal ileal–jejunal dilatation, with increase of gas–liquid stasis. Intraluminal tension is very high. Surgery revealed pelvic ileal bowel occlusion by fibrin

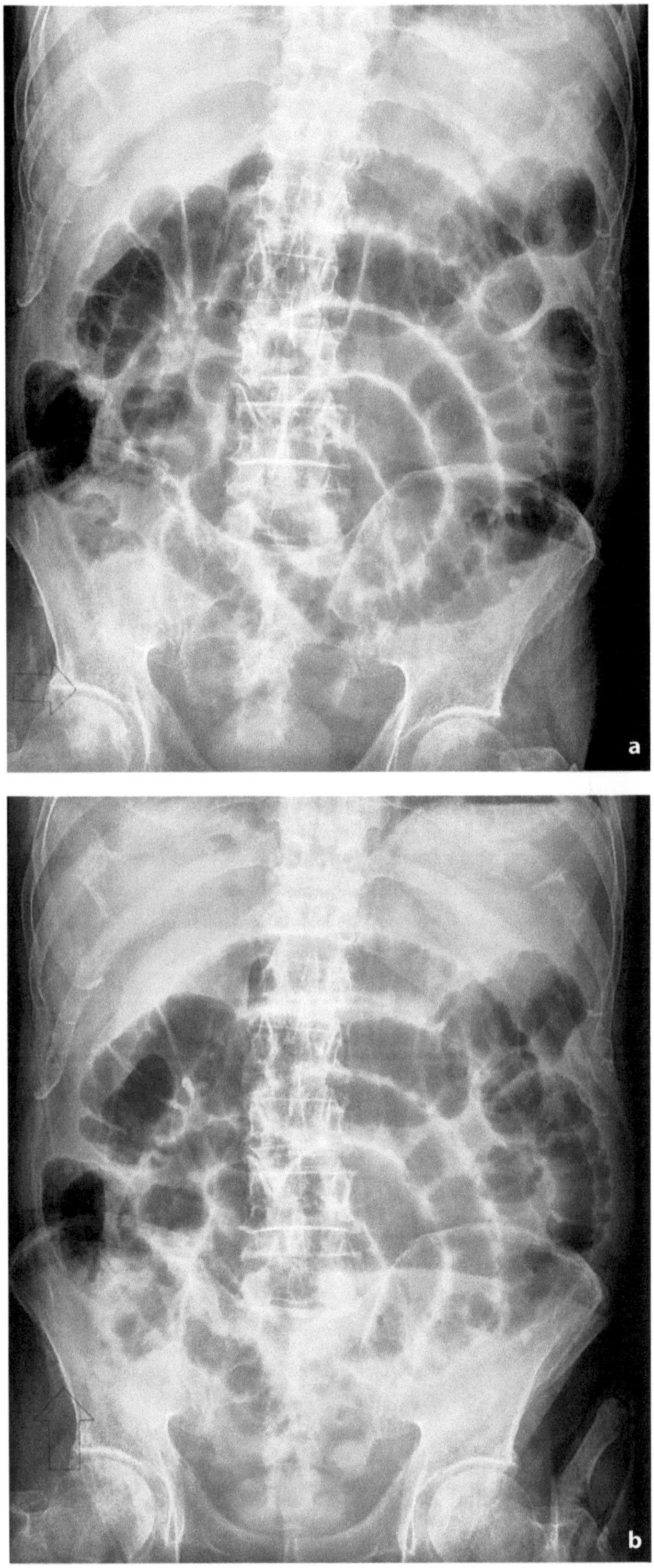

(cont. →)

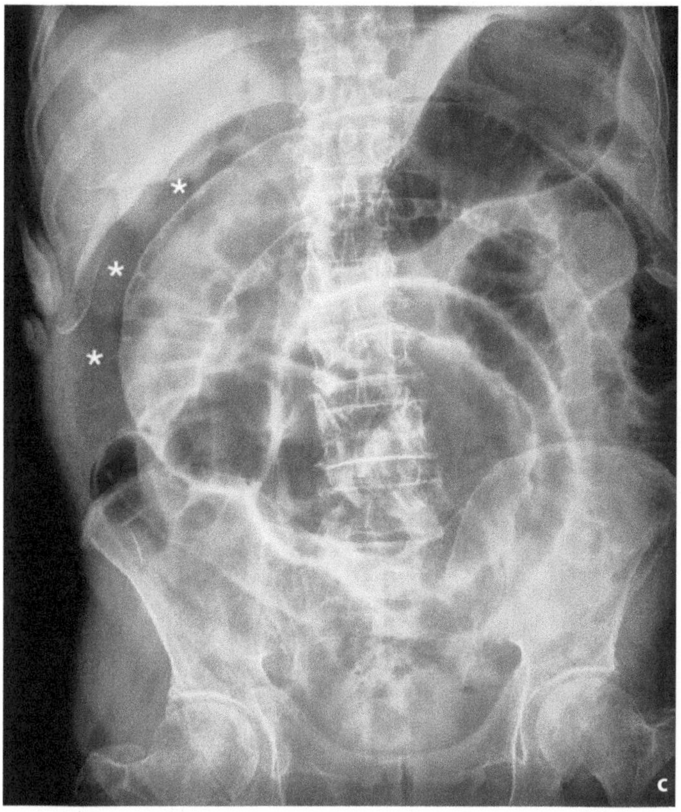

Fig. 5.19 a-c. Small-bowel obstruction (SBO) worsening. **a** Anteroposterior supine and **b** upright radiographs. SBO with massive distension. Anomalous loop location, which assumes a spiral configuration due to volvulus. Gas–liquid stasis. Right colon moderately represented. Initial intestinal-wall thickening due to vascular changes. Poor clinical condition of the elderly patient advised against surgical treatment. **c** Follow-up at 72 h. AP supine radiograph. The patient is not able to assume upright position. Presence of massive free peritoneal air (*asterisks*) is confirmed by Rigler's sign and the "bright liver". Absence of surgical intervention led to the final stage of acute intestinal ischaemia, with necrosis ⟹ perforation ⟹ peritonitis. Drastic tone decrease, with abnormal intestinal dilatation. Proximal jejunal loops show substantially preserved walls and valvulae. Other gas-containing ileal–jejunal segments show a marked wall thickening. Remarkable gastric ectasia, indicative of seriousness of the condition. Right colon poorly represented. Paralytic ileus due to peritonitis with perforation is superimposed to complicated SBO

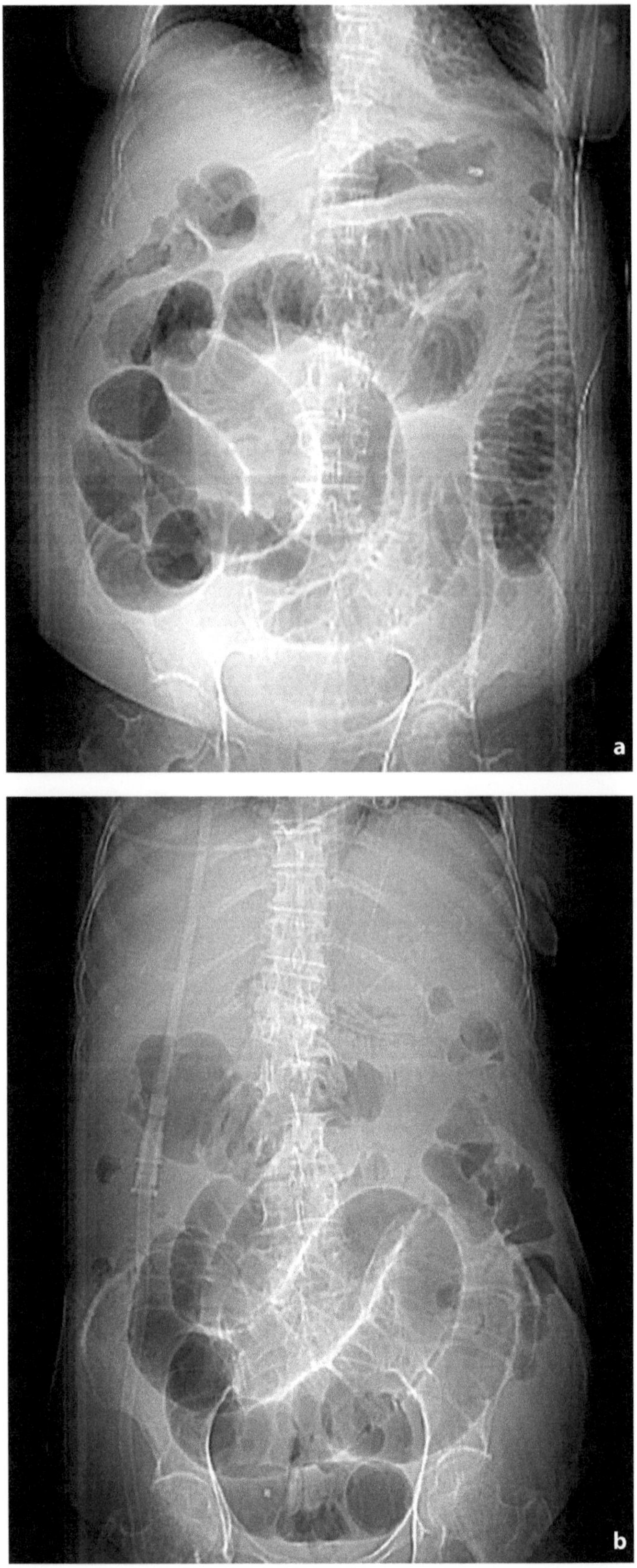

Fig. 5.20 a-d. Differential diagnosis between small-bowel mechanical ileus (MI) and paralytic ileus (PI). Every patient presented air–liquid levels on upright radiographs (not shown). **a, b** MI: anteroposterior supine radiographs of two patients. Presence of nasogastric tube. Interruption of luminal continuity causes increased intraluminal tension, which forces intestinal distension. Loops preserve characteristic tonic and curved aspect for a long period. Thin valvulae conniventes, with a crowded and forced appearance, are particularly evident. *(cont.* →)

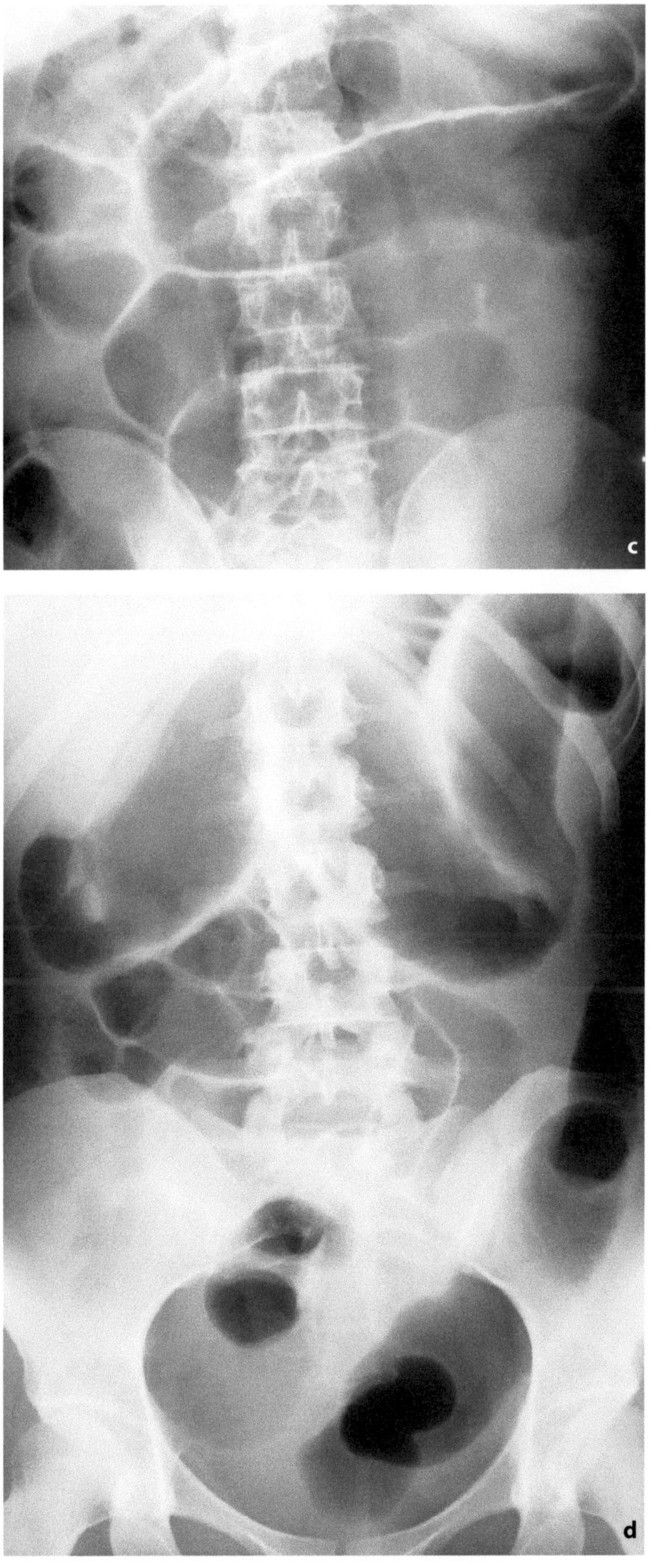

c, d Small-bowel PI. AP supine radiographs of two patients. Reduction of loop basal tone allows intestinal gas to expand and occupy all available space. Loops tend to be crowed in a rectilinear pattern. Absence of forced valvulae conniventes. No typical intraluminal tension of MI

Selected Readings

Amodio C, Antico E, Zaccarelli A et al (1991) L'esame radiografico diretto e l'ecografia dell'addome nella sindrome di occlusione intestinale. Radiol Med 81:286-292

Aufort S, Charra L, Lesnik A et al (2005) Multidetector CT of bowel obstruction: value of post-processing. Eur Radiol 15:2323-2329

Baker SR (1990) The abdominal plain film. Appleton and Lange, McGraw Hill, New York

Balthazar EJ, Birnbaum BA, Megibow AJ et al (1992) Closed-loop and strangulating intestinal obstruction: CT signs. Radiology 185:769-775

Bolondi L, Caletti G, Casanova P et al (1986) Problems and variations in the interpretation of the ultrasound feature of the normal upper and lower GI tract wall. Scand J Gastroenterol 21:16-26

Boudiaf M, Soyer P, Terem C et al (2001) CT evaluation of small bowel obstruction. Radiographics 21:613-624

Burkill G, Bell J, Healy J (2001) Small bowel obstruction: the role of computed tomography in its diagnosis and management with reference to other imaging modalities. Eur Radiol 11:1405-1422

Chou CK (2002) CT manifestations of bowel ischemia. AJR Am J Roentgenol 178:87-91

Delabrousse E, Destrumelle N, Brunelle S et al (2003) CT of small bowel obstruction in adults. Abdom Imaging 28:257-266

Di Mizio R, Merlini A (1992) L'addome a vuoto. In: Altaras J, Di Mizio R (eds) Nuovo atlante del colon e del tenue. Integrazioni di metodiche diagnostiche. Edizioni Libreria Cortina, Verona, pp 365-388

Di Mizio R, Grassi R, Marchese E et al (1995) Ileo meccanico 'scompensato' dell'intestino tenue nell'adulto. Rilievo ecografico di liquido libero tra le anse e suo significato prognostico. Radiol Med 89:787-791

Di Mizio R (2000) Occlusione meccanica dell'intestino tenue: radiologia-ecografia. In: Romano L (ed) L'addome acuto radiologico. Dal sintomo all'imaging. Idelson-Gnocchi, Napoli, pp 113-118

Fleischer AC, Bowling AD, Wienstein ML et al (1979) Sonographic patterns of distended fluid-filled bowel. Radiology 133:681-685

Frager DH, Baer JW (1995) Role of CT in evaluating patients with small bowel obstruction. Semin Ultrasound CT MR 13:127-140

Frassineti A (1997) Imaging diagnostico dell'ileo biliare. Imaging views. Editoriale Bracco, Milano

Frassineti A (1998) Imaging diagnostico della invaginazione intestinale. Imaging views. Editoriale Bracco, Milano

Frassineti A (2003-2005) Archivio radiografico tradizionale delle occlusioni meccaniche del tenue. CD n. 1-4. Editoriale Bracco, Milano

Furukawa A, Yamasaki M, Furuichi K et al (2001) Helical CT in the diagnosis of small bowel obstruction. Radiographics 21:341-355

Grassi R, Romano S, D'Amario F et al (2004) The relevance of free fluid between intestinal loops detected by sonography in the clinical assessment of small bowel obstruction in adults. Eur J Radiol 50:5-14

Grassi R, Di Mizio R, Pinto A et al (2004) Semeiotica radiografica dell'addome acuto all'esame radiologico diretto: ileo riflesso spastico, ileo riflesso ipotonico, ileo meccanico ed ileo paralitico. Radiol Med 108: 56-70

Griswold VJ (1999) Small bowel disease. Emergency Radiology 6:41-44

Ha HK, Rha SE, Kim JH et al (2000) CT diagnosis of strangulation in patients with small bowel obstruction: current status and future direction. Emergency Radiology 7:47-55

Horton KM, Fishman EK (2000) Normal enhancement of the small bowel: evaluation with spiral CT. J Comput Assist Tomogr 24:67-71

Kahi CJ, Rex DK (2003) Bowel obstruction and pseudo-obstruction. Gastroenterol Clin N Am 32:1229-1247

Khurana B, Ledbetter S, McTavish J et al (2002) Bowel obstruction revealed by multidetector CT. AJR Am J Roentgenol 178:1139-1144

Kim JH, Ha HK, Kim JK et al (2004) Usefulness of known computed tomography and clinical criteria for diagnosing strangulation in small bowel obstruction: analysis of true and false interpretation groups in computed tomography. World J Surg 28:63-68

Kimmey MB, Martin RW, Haggit RC et al (1989) Histological correlates of gastrointestinal ultrasound images. Gastroenterology 96:433-441

Lappas JC, Reyes BL, Maglinte DDT (2002) Abdominal radiography findings in small bowel obstruction. Relevance to triage for additional diagnostic imaging. AJR Am J Roentgenol 176:167-174

Ledermann HP, Borner N, Strunk H et al (2000) Bowel wall thickening transabdominal sonography. AJR Am J Roentgrnol 174:107-115

Lvoff N, Breiman RS, Coakley FV et al (2003) Distinguishing features of self-limiting adult small bowel intussusception identified at CT. Radiology 227:68-72

Macari M, Balthazar EJ (2001) CT of bowel wall thickening. Significance and pitfalls of interpretation. AJR Am J Roentgenol 176:1105- 1116

Macari M, Chandarana H, Balthazar EJ et al (2003) Intestinal ischemia versus intramural hemorrhage: CT evaluation. AJR Am J Roentgenol 180:177-184

Maglinte DDT, Herlinger H (1989) Plain film radiography. In: Herlinger H, Maglinte DDT (eds) Clinical radiology of the small intestine. Saunders, Philadelphia, pp 45-70

Maglinte DDT, Heitkamp DE, Howard TJ et al (2003) Current concepts in imaging of small bowel obstruction. Radiol Clin N Am 41:263-283

Maglinte DDT, Kelvin FM, Sandrasegaran K et al (2005) Radiology of small bowel obstruction: contemporary approach and controversies. Abdom Imaging 30:160-178

Makita O, Ikushima I, Matsumoto N et al (1999) CT differentiation between necrotic and nonnecrotic small bowel in closed loop and strangulating obstruction. Abdom Imaging 24:120-124

Okino Y, Kiyosue H, Mori H et al (2001) Root of the small bowel mesentery: correlative anatomy and CT features of pathologic conditions. Radiographics 21:1475-1490

Puylaert JB (2001) Ultrasound of acute GI tract conditions. Eur Radiol 11:1867-1877

Quiroga S, Alvarez-Castells A, Sebastià MC et al (1997) Small bowel obstruction secondary to bezoar: CT diagnosis. Abdom Imaging 22:315-317

Rha SE, Ha HK, Lee SH et al (2000) CT and MR imaging findings of bowel ischemia from various primary causes. Radiographics 20:29-42

Sandrasegaran K, Maglinte DDT, Howard TJ et al (2003) The multifaceted role of radiology in small bowel obstruction. Semin Ultrasound CT MR 29:319-335

Scaglione M, Romano S, Pinto F et al (2004) Helical CT diagnosis of small bowel obstruction in the acute clinical setting. Eur J Radiol 50:15-22

Scaglione M, Grassi R, Pinto A et al (2004) Valore predittivo positivo e valore predittivo negativo della TC spirale nella diagnosi di occlusione meccanica acuta ad ansa chiusa complicata da ischemia intestinale. Radiol Med 107:69-77

Suri S, Gupta S, Sudhakar PJ et al (1999) Comparative evaluation of plain films, ultrasound and CT in the diagnosis of intestinal obstruction. Acta Radiologica 49:422-428

Wiesner W, Khurana B, Ji H et al (2003) CT of acute bowel ischemia. Radiology 226:635-650

Wind P, Malamut G, Cuénod CA et al (2004) Stratégie des explorations des douleurs abdominales. EMC-Médecine 1:194-209

Wittenberg J, Harisinghani MG, Jhaveri K et al (2002) Algorithmic approach to CT diagnosis of the abnormal bowel wall. Radiographics 22:1093-1107

Zalcman M, Sy M, Donckier V et al (2000) Helical CT signs in the diagnosis of intestinal ischemia in small bowel obstruction. AJR Am J Roentgenol 175:1601-1607

Zissin R, Osadchy A, Gutman V et al (2004) CT findings in patients with small bowel obstruction due to phytobezoar. Emergency Radiology 10:197-200

MIX
Papier aus verantwortungsvollen Quellen
Paper from responsible sources
FSC® C105338

If you have any concerns about our products,
you can contact us on
ProductSafety@springernature.com

In case Publisher is established outside the EU,
the EU authorized representative is:
Springer Nature Customer Service Center GmbH
Europaplatz 3, 69115 Heidelberg, Germany

Printed by Libri Plureos GmbH
in Hamburg, Germany